D1217317

1818957
FO-C.

INTERVERTEBRAL DISCS AND OTHER MECHANICAL DISORDERS OF THE LUMBAR SPINE

EVIDENCE BASED CONSERVATIVE MANAGEMENT AND TREATMENT

C.K. Fernando: PhD, BSc, MA, FAAPM, MSCP, PT,
Executive Director of Forest Hills Institute for Back Pain, Inc.
and Island Rehabilitation Center

&

Dr. Arthur Nelson: PhD, FAPTA, Former Distinguished
Chairman of New York University, Professor of
Biology/Physical Therapy: University of New York City.

Authors Choice Press
New York   Bloomington

Intervertebral Discs and Other Mechanical Disorders of the Lumbar Spine
Evidence-Based Conservative Management and Treatment

Copyright © 2007, 2009 by C.K. Fernando.

Authors Choice Press
an imprint of iUniverse, Inc.

iUniverse books may be ordered through booksellers or by contacting:

iUniverse
1663 Liberty Drive
Bloomington, IN 47403
www.iuniverse.com
1-800-Authors (1-800-288-4677)

ISBN: 978-1-4401-3451-7 (pbk)

Printed in the United States of America

iUniverse rev. date: 3/23/2009

PREFACE

Ever since I began my clinical practice more than forty years ago, I've enjoyed working with patients. I've been particularly gratified to help them with their problems because, happily, they almost always get better.

Back pain is one of the most widespread and persistent of human maladies, even more common than the common cold. In the western world it is epidemic. In the U.S., 70-80% of the population will experience a back problem at some time in their lives. Back pain is the most common reason people miss work and the symptom most frequently brought to medical attention. It can severely limit sufferers' activities by curbing their ability to perform workday tasks and participate in sports.

What is more, back pain is the most expensive disease – not only to stricken individuals to whom the financial burdens are huge, but also due to lost workdays, to the industrial community where the economic costs are staggering. Human and social costs are enormous. Unfortunately, the high cost of care for patients with back pain creates additional problems of particular concern to physical therapists.

In the present climate of managed health care and government-issued systems, the main focus has shifted away from medical evidence and the patients' pathology. Instead, published treatment programs follow popular fashions and often impose restrictions designed to limit expenditures. Financial resources and availability of physicians and therapists may be major factors in determining protocols.

i

For instance, the Medicare program in the U.S. allowed only $1500 per patient for physical therapy regardless of pathology. This, obviously, was not based on clinical evidence. Similarly, the programs of the insurance industry exist primarily to control costs, hence are suspect. Health Maintenance Organizations strictly limit the numbers of treatments allotted for various problems and the choice of modalities as well. Furthermore, in countries with a socialist economy where medical care is dispensed by the state, medical insurance programs must take problems of finance and lack of physicians and therapists into account, hence scientific merit inevitably takes second place in their agenda.

Finally, to crown it all, the Quebec Task Force Report on Spinal Disorders, which was called a landmark in its time, seemingly legitimized these restrictions by jettisoning pathology-based diagnoses!

The public wants to believe that programs and guidelines issued by the government are reasonable, safe, and effective. The fact is that protocols developed by government edict exist primarily for the purpose of controlling costs and available manpower and not to adequately address patient welfare. Systems such as the one published by the Agency for Health Care Policy and Research (AHCPR) use criteria that have no basis in medical science and deserve no place in rational management.

Ironically, the emphasis on economics is counterproductive. The systems and therapies that supposedly save money by taking shortcuts leave many patients with lingering complaints. These patients will then miss more work because of back pain, and may go on to require surgery or become chronic back patients.

To spare patients the fate of chronic back problems and to lower the numbers of surgeries to more realistic levels, appropriate care is essential from the earliest stages on. Prompt, systematic, diagnoses must be made at the outset based on thorough clinical evaluations using modem techniques newly available to physical therapists. This must be followed by pathology-directed, conservative physical therapy based on scientific evidence; in short, the best treatments presently available for intervertebral disc disease and other mechanical disorders of the lumbar spine. In this way, most problems can be diagnosed and then resolved with excellent results.

The conservative modalities explained in this book exemplify such physical therapy. I developed these techniques at New York University Medical Center where I completed my Masters' thesis on treatment of low back pain and have practiced them since 1966. They are almost always successful in resolving my patients' back problems, so I can confidently, wholeheartedly, recommend them.

C.K.F.

ABOUT THE AUTHORS

Director of Forest Hill Institute for Back Pain, Inc. and the Island Rehabilitation Center, Dr. Fernando is a Fulbright Scholar and a graduate of New York University. While at NYU, he was a recipient of the Founders Award for Scholastic Achievement. Formerly an Assistant Professor of Physical Therapy at the College of Health Related Professions, Dr. Fernando is an international authority on back pain. Dr. Fernando has also served as: Associate Clinical Professor at the University of Illinois in Chicago, Director of Physical Therapy at Mt. Sinai Medical Center, Director of Physical Therapy at Schwab Rehabilitation Center and Director of Physical Therapy at Johnson R. Bowman Center. Dr. Fernando resides with his wife in Florida.

Dr. Arthur Nelson, Professor of Biology and Physical Therapy, College of Staten Island, City University of New York. Director of Clinical Research. Named distinguished professor of Physical Therapy at New York University, 2001. Invited Keynote Speaker, Asian World Confederation for Physical Therapy, 1999 Jakarta, Indonesia. Professor and Chairman, Physical Therapy Department, New York University. Post Doctoral Study: Biomechanics of Human Motion, Standord University, 1967. Dr. Nelson is a graduate of New York University where he was awarded the founders award for scholastic acheivement. He is a well known researcher, writer and lecturer and published many peer reviewed articles including the journal of Physical Therapy.

DEDICATION

To my wife, Laura Mahnil, whose love and support made this project possible, and to my daughters, Natasha and Tanya, and to my son Rajiv, whose constant encouragement has made this possible. Also, to my son-in-law Frank and my grandchildren, Anthony and Giana. As a cancer survivor, this major work stands as a testament to the resiliency of the human spirit.

C.K.F

ACKNOWLEDGMENTS

I am in debt to my former partner and associate, Sara Lane Harrer, MB A, OTR/L, without whom a first draft would have been impossible. My editor Rana Weiss, whose meticulous and careful work will make this, I'm sure, a great book. My assistant editor Sam Corbett, whose hard work was essential in transforming this book from first draft to final manuscript. Also, Terri Larner, my office manager, for her hard work in gathering and securing the necessary publishing permissions for the use of the diagrams and figures included herein.

C.K.F.

I must thank my "bride" of two years, Ardeth B Nelson, for proof reading and clarifying my contribution to this important book. My daughter, Susan Nelson Colaneri, was the department secretary at New York University when I was Chairman of the Physical Therapy department. It was during 1973 that Dr. Nelson developed the first doctor of Philosophy degree in Physical Therapy in the US. Since that time, forty-six Physical Therapists have been awarded the PhD Degree. Many thanks to my daughter, Susan N. Colaneri, who managed my Physical Therapy practice for fifteen years. Dr. Nelson is honored to be a contributor to this seminal work that outlines a most comprehensive review of effective care for those with lumbar pain syndromes.

A.J.N

vi

FOREWORD

Anyone who knows C.K. Fernando knows he is enthusiastic, dedicated and driven to perfecting anything useful. This book is a glowing example of that drive and experience. It should strengthen the hands and minds of several branches of the healing professions while clearing the debris of dubious techniques. Both teachers and practitioners must learn from its lessons.

– J.V. Basmajian, M.D.; D.Sc.
Professor Emeritus, McMaster University, Hamilton, Ontario.
Former Director, Emory University
Rehab Research & Training Center, Atlanta, Georgia.

TABLE OF CONTENTS

viii

x

I

EPIDEMIOLOGY

The study of how often a disease occurs and its distribution among various groups in the human population is essential in order to plan and evaluate strategies for prevention. And most importantly, epidemiology provides an understanding of the natural history of a disease so that treatments can be validated and their efficacy appraised.

Two relevant concepts are prevalence and incidence. Prevalence is a measure of the number of cases of a disease in a designated population at a particular time, while incidence is a measure of the rate at which new cases occur during a specified period. For instance, low back pain has a prevalence in a given year for a given population of approximately 5% while its incidence reportedly ranges from as low as 1% to as high as 20% per year depending on the specific population surveyed.[1]

Many studies inform us regarding both prevalence and incidence. However some, rather than being purely scientific, are designed to increase or decrease payment by insurance companies.

To better understand the short-term and long-term results and aftermath of back pain, we need new methods of studying its course and improved data on outcomes.[2] According to Saal[3], managed care of low back pain is based on the assumption that 90% of patients improve in 6-12 weeks. However, a natural history study by Van Korff[2] found that 60-75% improve in one

1

month, 33% report intermittent or persistent pain at the end of one year, and 20% of patients describe substantial limitations at one year. The premise of the AHCPR guideline and managed care for back pain is not valid.[3]

With these limitations in mind, a few natural studies of the lumbar spine, which are treated by physical therapists, are relevant. The National Health and Nutrition Examination (NHANE)[4] surveyed 10,404 civilians, non-institutionalized adults in the U.S. Of these, 1,355 had low back pain lasting more than two weeks and 5% had chronic symptoms lasting more than six months. Extrapolating the 5% with back pain to the current U.S. population of over 280 million yields a *total of over 14 million persons with chronic pain. Another 38,640,000 persons in the survey had* sciatica and low back pain, yielding a lifelong prevalence of 13.8%.[4]

Deyo[5] states that when patients' low back pain and leg pain persists for four weeks: 4-5% have symptoms of spinal stenosis, 4% have compression fractures, and 1% have a primary metastasis tumor or osteomylitis; fewer than 1% have a visceral disease, a renal condition, an aortic aneurism or gynecological problem.[5] Most studies agree that the 10% of patients with chronic low back pain account for 80-90% of the costs of health care for back pain.[6-8]

According to Nachemson[9], 85% of people with back pain lose fewer than seven days of work and account for about half the total workdays lost due to this malady. The other 15% of back pain sufferers stay at home for more than one month and account for the other half of workdays lost due to back pain. According to the National Health Interviews Survey of 30,074 workers in the U.S., about 22.4 million people, 17.6% of all U.S. workers, lost an estimated 149 million days from work as a result of back pain.[10]

DEFINITIONS OF LOW BACK DISORDERS

Low Back Pain. Unfortunately, the term low back pain is an inexact, catch-all category. Because the definition is not standardized, many studies of its prevalence, incidence and outcomes are not comparable. Adding to the confusion, studies performed for insurance purposes differ in methodology from those conducted for medical and scientific purposes. A better understanding of low back pain and its short-term and long-term outcomes must await more reliable data as our methods of studying the course of the disease improve.[11]

Sciatica is pain along the route of the sciatic nerve, often appearing as a motor or sensory deficit such as tingling, burning, or pins and needles; the anterior primary rami of one or more roots of the sciatic nerve, usually the L5, S1 and occasionally the S2, are involved. When the L4 and L3 nerve roots are involved, the femoral nerve is affected and the pain radiates down the anterior thigh.

The NHANE survey reported that 11% of the population has sciatica. The number of persons who can expect to get sciatica at some time during their lives has been variously estimated from 40% of adults to 13.8% of women and 22.4% of men between 45 and 54 years of age.[12]

Many studies show that sciatica is prevalent among those involved in heavy manual work.[13-16] Recent Finnish studies of sciatica in male concrete workers revealed a high prevalence rate of 42% and for those over 45 years of age, 60%.[17] Five years later, the lifetime prevalence had increased to 59% for all ages.[18,19] In the same studies, nurses and nurses' aides also showed high prevalence rates: 38% of nurses and 43% of nurses aides had experienced sciatica at least once. In contrast, only 5% of nursing school applicants, averaging 22.1 years of age reported a history of sciatica. A U.S. study found the highest prevalence of sciatica among adults 45 to 64 years of age.[20]

DURATION OF BACK DISEASE

In a survey of 10,404 non-institutionalized adults, 5% had backaches that had lasted for over six months.[21] Applying this rate to the entire U.S. population of 280 million, we would expect over 14 million persons to have chronic low back pain.

In the same survey, 1,355 individuals had low back pain that had lasted more than two weeks and an additional 161 had sciatica along with low back pain, making the total prevalence of low back pain 14.5%, and of sciatica, 1.5%.

Van Korff found that 60-75% of patients improve in a month; after a year, 33% report persistent or intermittent pain and 20% report substantial limitations.[23] The managed care system for primary care of back pain is based on the premise that 90% of patients improve in 6-12 weeks (42-84 days). So it appears that the guidelines of the Agency for Health Care Policy and Research (AHCPR) are based on an invalid premise according to Saal.[24]

DISABILITY DUE TO BACK PAIN

Although psycho-social factors may still be modifiers of pain, mechanical or idiopathic low back pain is likely to have its origins in pathology.[24, 25] The National Health Interview Survey of 30,074 workers (1995) indicated that 17.6% of all workers in the U.S., over 22 million people, lost an estimated 149 million work days because of back pain.[26] Nachemson states that 15% of patients with low back pain miss more than a month of work and

4

that these 15% account for half of the total number of workdays lost as a result of back pain.[27] According to this author, the remaining 85% lose a median of fewer than seven days of work.

RISK FACTORS FOR BACKACHE

Frequent lifting of heavy objects and twisting are risk factors for U.S. men 20-64 years of age. Kelsey, in a 1984 study, found other contributory factors to be time spent riding in motor vehicles (vibrations to the spine) and smoking.[28]

Heavy manual labor, lifting, twisting, driving (whole body vibration), monotonous work, low job satisfaction, poor physical fitness and smoking all are commonly related to back pain.

Some clinicians regard sitting as a risk factor. Sitting exerts more pressure on the disc at L3 than does standing, however the load is static and small compared to the amount required experimentally to cause damage.[29] Bigos found none of the studies on effects of sitting to be scientifically acceptable.[30]

SURGERY

A revealing study shows that the number of back surgeries increased by a surprising 49% during the period from 1979 to 1987. At the same time, the non-surgical hospitalizations for low back pain decreased by 33%.[31] The number of surgical procedures varied according to the region: in 1987, there were 77 surgeries per 100,000 adults in the northeast and 146 per 100,000 adults in the south. The authors attributed the discrepancy to cultural differences and patterns of practice.[31]

During a later period, from 1987 to 1990, Taylor et al. found an alarming rise in surgical interventions: surgeries for low back pain increased by 55%; fusions increased by 100%, from 13 to 26 per 100,000 adults and the more common surgical procedures also increased by 47% – from 89 to 131 per 100,000 adults.[32] At the same time that the number of surgeries rose, non-surgical hospitalizations decreased from 402 per 100,000 in 1979 to 150 per 100,000 in 1990.[32]

In 1990, the most recent year for which comparisons are available, the U.S. led thirteen other industrial nations in the number of surgeries for back pain with a rate 40% higher than any other country.[33] Again, the ever increasing numbers of surgeries are explained as due to cultural differences and practice patterns. These differences may well be inadequate therapy during the acute stages and of ineffective or even harmful non-surgical treatments such as mobilization, manipulation and unproven techniques of cults newly popular in the U.S.

Waddell, in a study that focuses mainly on the timing of surgical referrals and imaging, indicates that for the 1-2% of patients who need surgery this is important.[34] But as reported by Marcus in the Wall Street Journal in 2003, for the 95% or more with simple strains, sprains and nonspecific backache, surgery is inappropriate and can initiate or speed up the onset of arthritis.

Saal, in his 1996 presidential address to the North American Spine Society, pointed to flourishing fellowships with a "fix-it paradigm:" if disc excision doesn't work, there is fusion, and if that doesn't work, there is fusion revision with hardware and interbody grafts, and if that fails, the hardware can be removed and other options explored.[35] More recently, Frymoyer decried the initial enthusiasm for new fusion techniques; inevitably, the realization follows that these procedures do not solve the problems of disabilities. He laments, "When will we ever learn?"[36]

Another reason for the increase in spinal surgery may be the transfer of executive management of physical therapy to major corporations. This creates a conflict of interest for surgeons in their employ, since the more procedures they perform, the more their incomes increase. The Wall Street Journal of April 8, 2003, reported that Health South, a rehabilitation company based in Alabama, had revenues of 4.4 billion dollars in 2002. With 1700 facilities and 203 surgical centers, they had 900,000 surgical cases, and the revenue for the surgical centers for that year was 1 billion dollars. Health South had 3500 physician partners who received 49% of profits each quarter from the surgical center revenues. The physicians limited physical therapy patients to 14 visits, after which other treatment options such as epidural shots or surgery were initiated.

This method of operation is standard for all other publicly held rehabilitation corporations in the country. The American Physical Therapy Association is aware of this practice and is taking steps to curb these abuses.

What patients with back pain need is relief of pain, information, counsel, rehabilitation and preparation for going back to work. Clearly, the situation calls for a return to conservative standards of basic physical therapy practice: careful clinical evaluations including a complete history as in allopathic medical practice, diagnoses according to accepted pathology based criteria, and fundamental, tried and true treatments that do no harm to the patient and are appropriate to the diagnosis.

CHAPTER 1 NOTES

1. Borenstein DG, Wiesel SW, Boden SD. *Law Back Pain* 2nd ed. Philadelphia: WB Saunders; 1995: 22.
2. Von Korff M., Studying the natural history of back pain. *Spine*. 1994; (18S): 2045.
3. Saal JS. NASS Presidential Address. *Spine*. 1997; 22:1549.
4. Deyo RA, Tsui-Wu YJ. Descriptive epidemiology of low-back pain and its related medical care in the United States. *Spine*. 1987; 12: 264-268.
5. Deyo RA, Rainville J, Kent DL. *Neck and Back Pain*. Philadelphia; Lippincott-Raven; 1987:190.
6. Andersson G. The epidemiology of spinal disorders. In: Frymoyer J, Ed. *The Adult Spine: Principles and Practices*. New York: Raven Press; 1997: 93-141.
7. Johansson J, Ruvenowitz S. Risk indicators in the psychosocial and physical work environment for work-related neck, shoulder, and low back symptoms: A study among blue and white-collar workers in eight companies. *Scandinavian Journal of Rehabilitative Medicine*. 1994; 26: 131-142.
8. Nachemson A. Back pain in the workplace: A threat to our welfare states. In Wolter D, Seide K, Eds. *Berufsbedingte Erkrankungen der lenden'wirbelsaule*. Berlin: Springer-Verlag; 1998:191-206.
9. Nachemson A. *Back pain: Causes, Diagnosis, Treatment* (SBU Report). Stockholm: Swedish Council on Technology Assessment in Health Care; 1992.
10. Guo HR, Tanaka S, Cameron LL. Back pain among workers

in the United States: National estimates and workers at high risk. *American Journal of Industrial Medicine.* 1995; 28: 591-602.

11. Von Korff M. Studying the natural history of back pain. *Spine.* 1994;18S: 2041-2046.

12. Hirsch C, Jonsson B, Lewin T. Low-back symptoms in a Swedish female population. *Clinic of Orthopaedics.* 1969; 1: 171-176.

13. Wickstrom G, Hanninen K, Lehtinen M. Previous back syndromes and present back symptoms in concrete reinforcement workers. *Scandinavian Journal of Work Environment Health.* 1978; 4(Supplement I): 20-29.

14. Rihimaki H. Predictors of sciatic pain among concrete reinforcement workers and house painters: A five-year follow-up. *Scandinavian Journal of Work Environment Health.* 1989; 15:415-423.

15. Hrubed Z, Nashold BS Jr. Epidemiology of lumbar disc lesions in the Military in World War II. *American Journal of Epidemiology.* 1975; 102: 367-376.

16. Videman T, Nurimen T, Tola S. Low-back pain in nurses and some loading factors of work. *Spine.* 1984; 9: 61-66.

17. Wickstrom G, Hannimen K, Lehtinen M. Previous back syndromes and symptoms in concrete reinforcement workers. *Scandinavian Journal of Work Environment Health.* 1978; 4 (Supplement I): 20-29.

18. Nagi S, Riley LE, Newby LG. A social epidemiology of back pain in a general population. *Journal of Chronic Disease.* 1973; 26:769-779.

19. National Center for Health Statistics. *Prevalence of Selected Impairments.* DHHS Publication. 1981; No. 134: 81-1562.

20. Praemer A, Fumer S, Rice DP. *Musculoskeletal Conditions in the United States.* Park Ridge, DL: American Academy of

Orthopedic Surgeons; 1992.

21. National Center for Health Statistics. *Prevalence of Selected Impairments.* DHHS Publication. 1981; No. 134: 81-1562.

22. Frymoyer JW, Gordon SL. *New Perspectives on Low Back Pain.* Park Ridge, IL: American Academy of Orthopedic Surgeons; 1989.

23. Van Korff M. Studying the natural history of back pain. *Spine.* 1994; 18S: *2045S.*

24. Saal JS. NASS Presidential Address. *Spine.* 1997; 22: 1549.

25. Voliirn E, Lai D, McKinney S, et al. *When* back pain becomes disabling: A regional analysis. *Pain.* 1988; 33: 33-39

26. Guo HR, Tanaka S, Cameron LL. Back pain among workers in the United States: National estimates and workers at high risk. *American Journal of Industrial Medicine.* 1995; 28: 591-602.

27. Nachemson A. *Back pain: Causes, Diagnosis, Treatment.* (SBU Report) Stockholm: Swedish Council on Technology Assessment in Health Care; 1991.

28. Kelsey JL. An epidemiological study of the relationship between occupations and acute herniated lumbar intervertebral discs. *International Journal of Epidemiology.* 1978; 19:385-398.

29. Waddell G. *The Back Pain Revolution.* London: Churchill Livingstone; 1998.

30. *Bigos S. Reliable Science about Avoiding Law Back Problems at Work. Springer-Verlag; in press.*

31. Volinn E. Patterns in low back pain hospitalizations: Implications for the treatment of low back pain in an era of health care reform. *Clinical Journal of Pain.* 1994; 10: 64- 70.

32. Taylor VM, Deyo RA, Cherkin DC. Low back pain hospitalizations: Recent U.S. trends and regional variations. *Spine.* 1994; 19: 1207-1213.

33. Cherkin DC. Low back pain hospitalization: Recent United States trends and regional variations. *Spine.* 1994; 19: 1207-1213.

34. Waddell G. *The Back Pain Revolution.* London: Churchill Livingstone; 1998: 369-373.

35. Saal JS. NASS Presidential address. *Spine.* 1997; 22: 1549.

36. Frymoyer JW. Point of-view. *Spine.* 2001; 26: 747.

II

THE VERTEBRAL COLUMN

The vertebral column, or spine, is the central structural pillar of the body. Viewed from either the front or the back, it is straight. Viewed from the sagittal plane, it has four curves, two convex — the thoracic and the sacral, which bend back — and two concave — the cervical and the lumbar, which bend forward. In the cervical region, the vertebral column supports the head. In the lumbar region, it supports the entire trunk and this region is most frequently involved in backache.

Besides supporting the body, the vertebral column protects the spinal cord within the vertebral canal. See Figure 1.

FUNCTIONAL COMPONENTS OF THE VERTEBRAL COLUMN

The vertebrae, 33 bones stacked one on top of another, are similar in size and shape, the exception being the lumbar vertebrae, which are massive in comparison to the others. Between the vertebrae, cushioning them, are the intervertebral discs, which account for as much as a third of the height of the vertebral column. The discs, along with muscles and ligaments, connect the vertebrae to form a stable, strong and flexible column.

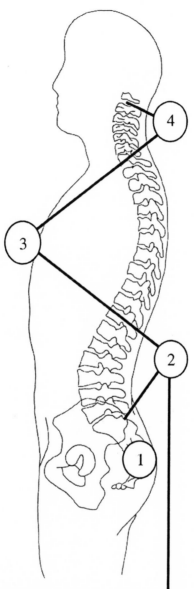

Viewed from the sagittal plane, it has four curves, two convex--the thoracic and the sacral which bend back--and two concave--the cervical and the lumbar which bend forward.

1,3--Sacral and Thoracic Convex

2,4--Cervical and lumbar Concave

Figure 1

The central portions of the vertebrae are called the vertebral bodies. Located behind them is the vertebral arch, which form a passageway, the vertebral foramen or spinal canal, which houses and protects the spinal cord. The spinal cord begins immediately behind and below the foramen magnum and ends at L1-L2 level as the conus madullaris. See Figure 2.

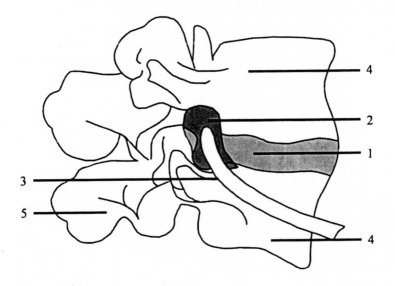

1 – Intervertebral Disc

2 – Intervertebral Foramen

3 – Spinal Nerve

4 – Vertebral Body

5 – Transverse process

Figure 2

THE VERTEBRAE

The 33 vertebrae — 7 cervical, 12 thoracic, 5 lumbar, 5 fused sacral and 4 coccygeal, are similar in basic design, but they increase in size and mass from the first cervical down to the last lumbar.

Structurally, a typical vertebra consists of two major parts:

1) *The vertebral body.* The anterior part is largest. It is wider than it is tall, cylindrical in shape and composed of cancellous bone covered by a thin shell of cortical bone. McBroom found that the vertebral cortices provided for only 10% of the total compressive load carried by the vertebrae.[1] In Osteoporosis, due to the loss of the horizontal trabecule, the vertical traberculae beams are weakened and hence the vertebral bodies are weakened. The superior and inferior surfaces of vertebral bodies, the end plates, are slightly concave.

2) *The vertebral arch*, the posterior part, a horseshoe-shaped projection, is attached to the vertebral body by two pedicles. Two laminae are situated posterior amid articular processes. The spinous process is posterior, attached at the midline, and the transverse processes are attached near the articular processes.

Intervertebral discs connect the vertebral bodies to each other. In addition, the articular process situated above one body, called a superior articular process, and the articular process situated beneath the body, called an inferior articular process, join to form a facet joint, or zyga pophysial joint. In this way, the vertebral bodies are joined in a column, forming a strong pillar to support the head and trunk.

Lumbar Vertebrae

Since the most common disorder of the spine is low back pain, the principle focus of this book is on the lumbar spine. The lumbar vertebrae support the entire trunk, as mentioned, and are massive compared to the other vertebrae. Their bodies are about 5 cm wide from side to side and 2 to 3 cm deep from front to back. Their lamina is broad, short and strong and their pedicles are very strong.

Largest in the lumbar region, the vertebral canal is approximately triangular, or trefoil shaped and decreases in size in the thoracic region, and is smallest in the cervical region.

The spinous process of a lumbar vertebra is thick and broad. The facets on the superior articular processes are concave and directed medially backward. The facets on the inferior processes are convex and directed laterally forward. The inferior and superior facets on the pedicles of adjacent vertebrae form the facet joints, which allow flexion, extension and side-to-side bending. If they allow any rotation at all, it is very minimal. Lumbar vertebrae have long and thin transverse processes.

The vertebral body L-5 is wedge-shaped, making it higher anteriorly than posteriorly. The basic design of vertebrae from C3 through L5 is similar, but from LI through L5 their size and mass increase to accommodate the increased compression loads to which they are subjected.

THE INTERVERTEBRAL DISCS

The intervertebral discs account for up to 33% of the height of the vertebral column and aid in load-bearing and shock absorption. Their geometry and physiological condition largely determine the biomechanical functioning of the vertebral column. A disc is composed of upper and lowers cartilaginous end plates and, sandwiched in between, a cartilaginous annulus fibrosus with a gelatinous center, the nucleus pulpous.

The end plates, 1 mm thick, consist of laminae of hyaline cartilage. They are avascular and relatively impermeable to molecules of large molecular weight, and thus form a barrier between the vascular spongiosa of the vertebral body and the avascular disc.[2]

Between the end plates, connecting them, are peripheral rings of lamellae-like fibrous cartilage, **the annulus fibrosus.** The annulus is made up of concentric layers of parallel fibers at a 45-degree angle to the vertebral bodies, forming a strong connection between them. These fibers present within the lamellae minimize any rupture of the annulus.

In general, the annulus consists of water, collagen, proteoglycan and, interspersed among the collagen fibers, chondrocytes and fibroblasts, which aid in synthesizing collagen and proteoglycan.

New studies, such as the one performed by Marchand, indicate the annulus has 15-25 laminae depending on age and the area of the spine.[3] About 40% of the layers, most of them in the postero-lateral area, are incomplete. Hence annular ruptures are more often seen in the postero-lateral region.

Within the annulus fibrosus is a central homogenous, semi gelatinous region, *the nucleus pulposus*, the largest avascular structure in the body. It is 70-90% water, 15-20% collagen and 5% proteoglycan. The water content decreases with age. Embedded in the proteoglycan are cartilage cells, responsible for synthesis of the proteoglycan and collagen of the nucleus pulposus.

Both the annulus and the nucleus have a large matrix of extra cellular components, namely collagen and proteoglycan. At birth, the water content of the annulus is about 80% and of the nucleus, 90%.[4] By the third decade of life, the water content of the annulus has decreased to 70% and of the nucleus, to 75%. Thereafter, the water content of the annulus remains at 70%, and that of the nucleus becomes about the same as the annulus.[4]

Vemon-Roberts reports that by middle age, the nucleus has lost its soft structure due to encroachment of collagen from the inner layers of the annulus.[5] Also, as a result of advanced age and disc protrusion, the protein-polysaccharide content of the nucleus decreases, reducing the thickness of the disc and thereby lowering its shock-absorbing capacity.[6]

The nucleus and the annulus are alike in many respects. Both consist of water, collagen and proteoglycan, but in different proportions. The nucleus consists mainly of water, proteoglycan and predominantly type II collagen, while the annulus consists of water, proteoglycan and large amounts of type II collagen as well as type I.

New studies indicate there are more than a few types of collagen in the annulus fibrosus. Nerlich ET al.[7] has now identified well over eight types of collagen in the human annulus – they being: Type I, II, III, IV, V, VI, IX, XI. They however noted both inter-individual and intra-individual variability in humans.

New findings by Nerlich[7] indicate that types I and II collagen occupy a three-dimensional location in the annulus, which is of clinical significance.

Type I collagen, composing the bulk of collagen in the annulus, is seen abundantly in the outer zone of the annulus, and the outer lamellas of the inner zone of the annulus fibrosus. The three-dimensional shape of type I collagen in the annulus is a donut-shape, wider anteriorly than posteriorly. This supports the view that the posterior section of the annulus in humans is weaker than the anterior section. This view is further strengthened by the fact that there are twice as many posterior disc bulging and protrusion incidences than anterior bulging.[7, 8]

If the proteoglycan core in the nucleus is destroyed (as in chymopapain treatment), the water-binding capacity of the disc is lost, lowering intra discal pressure.

In early 1951, Smith et al. showed that in a rabbit model the disc healed only in the superficial layers after incisions of its annulus were made.[9] In another study, Lipson and Muir[10] showed similar findings. According to them, due to initial defect in the annulus, for example when the annulus is punctured with a 20-gauge needle, only a small scar was found at the site of the needle track. Cutting the annulus with a knife leads to disc degeneration. There is an increase in aggregating proteoglycans at three weeks; this is an attempt to repair the annulus. Proliferation of the cells of the annulus could potentially seal off the defect in the annulus and restore a confining structure to the nucleus. But according to these authors this repair is never successful and results in mechanical failure.

A study by Hampton et al.[11] showed that in dogs, following surgically induced damage to the annulus, there formed two kinds of lesions: full thickness tissue blocks removed down to nucleus and stab wounds from annulus to nucleus pulposus. Gross and microscopic examination revealed that after nine weeks there was complete healing involving fibrous connective tissue when the tissue blocks were removed. They also found a formation of a fibrous pedicle cap at stab wound sites. They concluded that the stab wound sites were much like herniation sites, in that minor leakage of nuclear material causes chemical radiculitis and pain.

Another study by Ahlgren et al.[12] concluded that in sheep the early response of the disc after injury (up to 2-4 weeks) is loss of integrity involving pressurization and biomechanical stability when compared with controls. They also concluded that further healing (between 4-6 weeks) improves biomechanical properties considerably, as well as the ability to withstand internal pressurization. They also found that in the early healing phase, a box injury through the annulus causes significantly greater loss of annular integrity and a greater increase in motion segment flexibility than does a slit injury. A slit incision will seal the outer aspect of the annulus in a stronger manner than the box injury, especially in the early healing stages. See Figure 3.

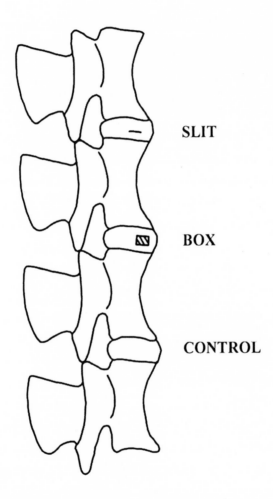

SLIT

BOX

CONTROL

Illustration of anular incisions made on anterolateral aspect of disc

Figure 3

These studies are the reason why therapists should explain to patients with disc herniations that they will heal if properly treated by the therapists; keeping intra discal pressures low so that no leakage of the pulposus will take place, thereby minimizing pain and also allowing the natural healing process to take place. In addition, it's also important to teach patients proper ADL techniques, so that they minimize intra discal pressure during activities. Any modality that helps in the disc healing process should be used, and the senior authors believe that Cortrel traction techniques, in combination with Ultrasound (US), Low Level Laser Therapy (LLLT) and Interferential Therapy (IT), are suitable ways to enhance healing of the annulus. It is also important in the acute and sub acute stages that stabilization exercises are done on stable surfaces (not Swiss balls!) so that intra discal pressures are kept as low as possible. All exercises are done within pain tolerance, so pain sensitive structures are not irritated so that the healing process will move forward without exacerbation.

One has to be aware of the intra discal pressures on the lumbar spine in various motions to appreciate what can be done with patients in therapy as well as in ADL.

THE INTERVERTEBRAL FORAMEN (IVF)

The intervertebral foramen (IVF) is bounded laterally, above and below, by the pedicles of adjacent vertebra. Anteriorly, it is bounded by the posterior borders of the intervertebral discs and adjoining parts of the vertebral bodies. Posteriorly, it is bounded by the articular processes and facet (zyga pophysial) joints, which are closely attached to the capsular ligament and bridged by the ligament flavum. Hoyland compares the cross-sectional shape of the IVF to that of an inverted pear.[13]

The nerve complex, situated at the upper pole of the foramen and occupying about 35% of its-cross-sectional area, consists of

21

nerve roots, dorsal root ganglia and the spinal nerve. Ordinarily, the IVF is spacious enough to accommodate these neural strictures so that direct compression of the nerve root is unlikely unless a gross amount of the disc protrudes.[14] In 42 cases of poster lateral disc herniations, only eight (19%) had identifiable compression of the nerve root, yet all showed peri-neural fibrosis.[14]

Marchand observed pathologic changes in nervous tissue in the IVF in association with disc protrusions that compress veins, leading to venous stasis and ischemia.[15] These authors suggest that improving venous drainage may be therapeutic.

Osteophytes that are postero-lateral in relation to the IVF can, either alone or along with prolapsed disc material, produce pressure on the spinal nerves causing symptoms similar to those caused by disc prolapse. Osteophytes from the margins of osteo-arthritic facet joints that impinge on the IVF can also cause similar symptoms. See Figures 8, 9 and 10.

As the nerve root emerges from the IVF in the lumbar and sacral area, the sinu-vertebral nerves arise as branches from each spinal nerve just distal to the DRG, then run back medially into the vertebral column through the IVF to be distributed to such structures as the posterior longitudinal ligament, ligamentum flava and posterior dura.[16]

Inufusa et al. found that during flexion the cross-sectional area of the foramen increased by 12.7 sq mm (11.8%).[17] Extension, on the other hand, produced a decrease in all dimensions of the foramen: the middle foramenal width and the foramenal cross-sectional area decreased by 0.9 sq mm (-20.9%) and 18.7 sq mm (-15.3%) respectively. Nerve-root compression was seen in 10 out of 50 cases (20%). In these subjects, a pre-loading nerve-root compression of 23.1% decreased after flexion-loading to 11.5%. A pre-loading nerve-root compression of 16.7% increased after extension loading to 37.5%. Posterior bulging of discs coupled with traction spurs significantly affected both flexion and extension.[17]

THE LATERAL LUMBAR SPINAL CANAL

The lateral lumbar spinal canal is a tubular canal from which the nerve root exits the IVF, consists of the nerve root canal, or lateral recess, and the IVF. The lateral lumbar spinal canal has three zones: the entrance, the midzone and the exit. The entrance is the subarticular region, also called the lateral recess area; the midzone is situated under *the pars intercularis*; and the exit is the IVF. According to Ciric et al., the height of the lateral recess is 5 mm or more; a height of 2 mm or less is pathologic and 3-4 mm is a cause for lateral spinal stenosis, which can cause lumbar radicular symptoms.[18]

Bose found that due to the slant of the lumbar roots, their canals have different lengths. The sacral canals also differ: the first is 3.5 mm long and the fourth, 2.5 mm. In the foramina for L5 and L4, the nerve roots occupy only one third of the vertical height; the rest of the space accommodates the facets during extension of the lumbar spine.[19]

In understanding the movements of intra discal dye in flexion and extension, Brock et al. studied 53 normal segments of lumbar spine and 47 segments of abnormal spines. Their conclusions were no changes in the abnormal spines, but movements in the normal subjects. If extension exercises are beneficial, the mechanism is independent of nuclear shift and may be related to gait theory, disc hydration or neural tissue relaxation. They found no changes in the position of the herniated disc through MRI before or after McKenzie Treatments.

In 2007, Alexander et al., showed by using MRI in different

functional positions; "prone extension, a posture commonly used as a treatment technique in physical therapies, induced significantly less posterior migration than any of the 3 sitting positions." Hence it is apparent that the McKenzie treatment rationale is invalid.[21]

Studies by Punjabi et al. clearly show that in flexion the size of the intervertebral foramen increased, while in extension the size decreased. In the normal spines the intervertebral foramen was 185 mm2. The intervertebral foramen was 24% larger in flexion, while in extension it was 20%. There were changes in the intervertebral foramen both in lateral bending and rotation, but they were less significant. This study has implications in treatment by physical therapy. For patients with disc herniations or spinal stenosis, its best to teach exercises in non pain-free situations, as pain is an indicator that either in flexion or extension the spinal nerve is compressed, causing pain and or paresthesia.[20]

CHAPTER 2 NOTES

1. McBroom, FJ Prediction of vertebral body compressive fracture using quantitative computed topography. *Journal of Bone and Joint Surgery.* 1985; 67A: 1206.

2. Bailey AJ, Herbert CM, Jayson M. Collagen of the Intervertebral Disc. Rpt in: Jayson M, ed. *Lumbar Spine and Back pain.* London: Pitman Medical Publishing Company; 1976: 328.

3. Marchand F, Ahmed AM. Investigation of the laminate structure of lumbar disc annulus fibrosis. *Spine.* 1990; 15: 410.

4. Vernon-Roberts B. Pathology of degenerative spondylolysis. In: Jayson M, ed. *Lumbar Spine and Back Pain.* London: Pitman Medical Publishing Company; 1976: 57.

5. Vernon-Roberts B. Pathology of degenerative spondylolysis. In: Jayson M, ed. *Lumbar Spine and Back Pain.* London: Pitman Medical Publishing Company; 1976: 57.

6. Vernon-Roberts B. Pathology of degenerative spondylolysis. In Jayson M, ed. *Lumbar Spine and Back Pain.* London: Pitman Medical Publishing Company; 1976: 58.

7. Nerlich AG, et al. Immunohistological markers for the age-related changes of human lumbar intervertebral discs. *Spine.* 1997; 22; 2781-95.

8. Schollmeier G, et al. Observations on fiber forming collagens in the annulus fibrosus. *Spine.* 2000; 25: 2736-2741.

9. Smith JW, et al. Experimental incision of the intervertebral disc. *Journal of Bone and Joint Surgery.* 1951; 33B: 612-625

10. Lipson SJ, Muir H. Proteoglycans in experimental intervertebral disc degeneration. *Spine.* 1981; 6:194-210,

11. Hampton D, Laros G, McCarron R, Franks D. Healing potential of annulus fibrosus. *Spine.* 1989;14; 398-401.

12. Ahlgren BD, Vasavada A, Brower RS, Lyndon C, Herkowitz HN, Punjabi MM. Annular incision technique on the strength and multidirectional flexibility of the healing intervertebral disc. *Spine.* 1994;19:953-54.

13. Hoyland JA, Freemont AJ, Jayson MIV. Intervertebral foramen venous obstruction: a cause of periradicular fibrosis? *Spine.* 1989; 14: 560.

14. Hoyland JA, Freemont AJ, Jayson MTV. Intervertebral foramen venous obstruction: a cause of periradicular fibrosis? *Spine.* 1989; 14: 566.

15. Marchand F, Ahmed AB. Investigation of the laminate structure of lumbar disc annulus fibrosis. *Spine.* 1990; 15: 402-410.

16. Wyke B. Neurological aspects of low back pain. In: Jayson M, ed. *Lumbar Spine and Back Pain.* London: Pitman Medical Publishing Company; 1976.

17. Inufusa A, An HS, Lim TH, et al. Anatomic changes of the spinal canal and intervertebral foramen associated with flexion-extension movement. *Spine.* 1996; 21: 2415

18. Ciric I, Mikhael MA, Tarkmgton JA, Vick NA. The later recess syndrome: A variant of spinal stenosis. *Journal of Neurosurgery. Spine.* 1980; 53: 433-443.

19. Bose K, Balasubramaniam P. Nerve root canals of the lumbar spine. *Spine.* 1984; 9:16.

20. Punjabi MM, Takata K, Goel VK. Kinematics of the lumbar intervertebral foramen. *Spme.19S3;* 8:348.

21. Alexander L, et al. The Response of the Nucleus Pulposus of the Lumbar Intervertebral Discs to Functionally Loaded Positions. Spine. 2007; 32; 1508-12

III

MUSCLES AND LIGAMENTS OF THE LUMBAR SPINE

The spine and its supporting and stabilizing musculo-ligamentous structures form the central machine that powers the body's movements and actions. The movements of the spine are: flexion, extension, lateral flexion and rotation. The chief activators of these movements are the muscles of the lumbar spine, which are contractile elements of stability and motion.

During movements and loading, co-activation of anterior and posterior spinal muscles appears to provide stability, according to Moshe.[1] Various spinal ligaments also play a minor part in stabilizing the spine during ordinary activities, as studies of White and Punjabi clearly show.[2] The ligaments function primarily as sensory receptors, monitoring movements and activating muscles via spinal neurons to restore and maintain stability, according to Moshe.[3] Upon mechanical deformation of the spinal ligament, the ligament invokes mechano-receptors in the supra-spinal ligament, which in turn activates the para-spinal muscles within the two rostra- and caudal-motion segments up to the point of the deformation of the ligament; this muscle activity stabilizes the lumbar spine.[4] Moshe concludes that strengthening the muscles improves stability and prevents injury to the lumbar spine. The senior

27

author agrees, having advocated this reasoning since 1967, and presented a paper to that effect at the 7th World Confederation of Physical Therapists in Montreal in 1974.[5]

In addition to controlling the biomechanics of daily activities, the spinal muscular framework also prevents injury of key joints such as the shoulder, and nerves including the peripheral nerve roots.[6]

The spinal mechanism is susceptible to overload, and chronic repetitive overload injuries. In persons whose occupations involve sustained activity, paraspinal muscles are subject to fatigue, which results in loss of stability of the spine; hence, these muscles and the ligaments around the lumbar spine are apt to be injured, when there is a loss of dynamic muscle protection. Many people in our industrial society are injured at work. In athletic activities, too, where trunk control and stability are essential to maximum efficiency and optimal performance, injuries are common.[7] Both in the workplace and in sports, most of these injuries are muscle strains and ligamentous sprains.

Physical therapists, to whom the study of muscles and ligaments is paramount and to whom this book is addressed, treat most of these patients. The muscles and ligaments that directly affect the stability of the lumbar spine are described in this chapter. For those not directly related to spinal function, readers are referred to other anatomy textbooks.

POSTERIOR MUSCLES OF THE TRUNK

A spine with its ligaments isolated and fixed at its base would collapse under a force of only 4.5 lbs. It does not collapse due to the support of two systems, namely the extrinsic and intrinsic stabilizers.[8]

(1) **The extrinsic stabilizers** are all the muscles surrounding the lumbar spine, including the abdominal and back extensor muscle groups, the lateral muscles and the iliopsoas.

(2) **The intrinsic stabilizers** are the ligaments around the lumbar spine and intra-abdominal pressures.

To improve these systems and enhance stability of the lumbar spine, this senior author has advocated the following physical therapeutic measures[9]: (A) strengthening the abdominal muscles; (B) strengthening the back extensor muscles; (C) strengthening the iliopsoas group. By strengthening the iliopsoas group, the extrinsic stabilizers are strengthened. In addition to this, the fact that this group of muscles weaken in patients with low back pain indicates that this procedure is necessary. Strengthening these three groups of muscles strengthens the intrinsic stabilizers, namely the intra-abdominal muscles. Weak muscles are more prone to develop spasm and therefore pain. In the treatment of low-back pain due to intervertebral disc lesions, when the acute episode subsides, exercise therapy may be commenced. The aim of treatment is to minimize intradiscal pressures by using non weight-bearing positions and pain-free ranges. This is important as a rise in intradiscal pressure in patients with herniation could lead to protrusion of the nucleus pulposus, which in turn could impinge on the sinuvertebral nerve or its branches, which innervate the posterior longitudinal ligament, the outer layer of the annulus, and the synovial joints, thereby giving rise to the pain and its resulting clinical syndrome. Nearly 50% of all intervertebral disc lesions are posterior, and only 10-12% are postero-lateral; these lesions could give rise to a radiating type of pain in the lower extremities.

In addition to this, the aim of treatment is to give stability to the lumbar spine so that repetitions of herniation, irritation, pain, and muscle spasms can be avoided.

Eie[10] studied the load capacity and intra-abdominal pressure in humans. He concluded that the intervertebral discs and their end plates withstood greater forces than the vertebrae themselves. He also concluded that 40% of intra-abdominal pressure was due to contraction of the erector spinae muscles.

Fernando[11] studied the extensor-flexor ratio of the trunk musculature quantitatively.

Using a dynamometer of the Cybex Exerciser System, the testing being done in the Clarke's sitting position, it was found that in normal subjects with no history of back pain, the extensor strength was always greater than the flexor strength for males and females. The mean extensor-flexor ratio was 1.5. In patients with chronic low back pain, the extensor-flexor ratio was .9

The Extrinsic Stabilizers

The extrinsic stabilizers bear directly on the stability of the spine. They may be divided into three categories: (1) posterior muscles of the trunk, (2) muscles of the abdominal wall, (3) lateral muscles of the trunk: quadratus lumborum and psoas.

Extension of the spine is the main function of the posterior muscles of the trunk, also called the back extensors. All the posterior muscles of the trunk lie behind the plane of the transverse processes. Bogduk and Twomey[12] subdivide them into three groups: (1) intersegmental muscles, (2) polysegmental muscles and (3) the latissimus dorsi, muscles which attach via the massive lumbo-dorsal fascia.

THE INTERSEGMENTAL MUSCLES

The intersegmental muscles are the inter-spinals and the inter-transversarii medialis. **The inter-spinals** are four short paired muscles on either side of the interspinous ligament, attached to the spinous processes.

The intertransversarii medialis are true back muscles innervated by the lumbar dorsal ramii from C1 and C2 through sacral roots. These muscles are densely endowed with muscle spindles and act as proprioceptive transducers, monitoring the movements of the lumbar spine and influencing the actions of the surrounding muscles.[13]

THE POLYSEGMENTAL MUSCLES

The polysegmental muscles attached directly to the lumbar vertebrae are the multifidus and the remaining lumbar erector spinae muscles. The **multifidus** is the most medial and largest of the back muscles. Most anatomy books designate as back muscles those attached to spinal structures. However, as Macintosh has clearly shown, the multifidus is extensively attached to both the sacrum and the iliac crest, and bridges the sacroiliac joint.[14] The multifidus acts by pulling downward on each spinous process it attaches to, extending the vertebra from which the muscle originates. The muscles are like fasciculi inserted into the maxillary processes below — sometimes 3 to 5 levels below — the origin. However, fibers from the L5 vertebra attach to the iliac crest and the posterior surface of the sacrum.

Chowlewick shows that in healthy persons, antagonistic trunk flexor-extensor muscles coactivate around the neutral spinal posture.[15] In lay terms, the muscle does double duty, hence it is susceptible to injury in athletes, workers and postsurgical patients. Persons with back pain show reduced muscle mass in the multifidus and significant wasting of both the erector spinae and the psoas muscles.[16] Stokes et al.[16] report a significant change in

31

dimensions of the multifidus on the side ipsilateral to radicular pain. They point out that its greater percentage of Type I over Type II fibers gives the multifidus a greater role in stabilizing the lumbar spine due to the Type I fibers' fatigue-resistance.[16] Spinal instabilities cause low back pain, and the principal role of the multifidus is to act as a segment-by-segment stabilizer of the spine. But according to Pope and Stokes et al., the precise role of the multifidus in spinal instabilities is unclear.[17, 18]

Anatomy textbooks call the multifidus a rotator of the lumbar spine, but this is not accurate. During spinal rotation, the main action of the multifidus is a rocking-like extension of the lumbar spine to oppose the flexion effect of the external and internal oblique abdominal muscles which actually produce the rotation. The multifidus, in this way, stabilizes the lumbar spine during rotation by co-contracting with the oblique abdominals.

Another effect of the multifidus is to increase the lumbar lordosis. This bowstring effect is a consequence of its being polysegmental. An experienced clinician recognizes the "flat-back" as a weak back because the lordosis is not formed due to insufficient multifidus action.

The lumbar erector spinae are the large dorsolateral muscles that can be seen lying laterally with respect to the multifidus muscle. They form a superficially tendinous muscle mass originating from the sacrum, iliac crest and the spinous processes of all the lumbar vertebrae and the last two thoracic vertebrae; hence the former name, sacro spinalis. There are three parts: (1) the iliocostalis lumborum — the most lateral— (2) the longissimus lumborum — the intermediate— and (3) the spinalis — the medial.

The fibers of the iliocostalis lumborum muscle arise from the very tips of the transverse processes of the L1-L4 vertebrae. Some also arise from the thoracolumbar fascia and insert into the tips of the transverse processes. Some of the fibers pass from these origins as flat sheets and insert into the crest of the ileum. They pull downward and backward on the transverse processes, thereby extending the lumbar vertebrae to minimize flexion. Acting unilaterally, they control lateral bending of the lumbar spine.

The longissimus thoracic pars lumborum muscle lies immediately lateral to the multifidus. It originates from the tips of the L1-L4 accessory processes and inserts into the ileum just medial to the posterior superior iliac spine. Its insertion is via a common tendon known as the lumbar intramuscular aponeurosis. Its action is the same as that of the iliocostalis lumborum pars lumborum.

These muscles, it must be remembered, are innervated by the dorsal ramii of the spinal nerves, except that a few in the lumbar region, the lateral intertransversarii for example, are innervated by the ventral ramii.

The erector **spinae aponeurosis** is a broad, flat tendon covering the posterior aspect of the lumbar region. It simply covers the underlying muscles in the lumbar region from medial to lateral, the longissimus thoracic pars lumborum and iliocostalis lumborum pars lumborum. However, the flat tendon of the aponeurosis is composed of the caudal tendons of the bellies of the muscles of the thoracic region, namely the longissimus thoracic pars thoracic and the iliocostalis lumborum pars thoracic.

The main action of the posterior muscles of the back, the back extensors, is extension of the spine. In addition, these muscles are active during flexion movements of the anterior muscles. And they strongly contract to control flexion movements which are mainly powered by gravity. On full flexion, however, the back extensors are electrically silent (the flexion-relaxation response). Bogduk et al.[19] demonstrated that thoracic fibers of the longissimus thoracic and iliocostalis lumborum manage over half of all extension in the lumbar area and the lumbar fibers of the same muscles and the multifidus manage the remainder of the movement. In the upright position, the multifidus and lumbar parts of the longissimus and iliocostalis exert posterior shear forces, mainly on L1-L4, and also anterior shear force on L5 due to the shape of the lumbar lordosis and the lumbosacral angle. On flexion, the lumbar lordosis is reduced thereby, the spine is straightened and the posterior shear forces on the upper lumbar vertebra are reduced.

The back muscles contribute little to axial rotation movements, at most 5% of maximum torque exerted during trunk rotation.[20]

Some authorities believe that the thoracic portion of the back extensors are the most efficient since they have the largest moment arm and greatest mechanical advantage as they course over the lumbar region. The vertebrae of the thoracic spine permits more rotation than the lumbar.

Stuart McGill correctly warns against exercises that challenge the lumbar muscles in isolation.[21] Such exercises are not justified from either an anatomic or a motor control standpoint. This senior author agrees, and for this reason recommends isometric back extension exercises, having proposed them as early as 1970.[22]

According to McGill, the lumbar sections of the longissimus and iliocostalis muscles create extensor torque due to their attachment to the lumbar vertebrae.[23] These muscles also produce great posterior shear forces to support the spine during flexion movements. McGill cautions therapists not to teach patients to deactivate these forces by practicing the pelvic tilt during lifting actions from flexed positions.

Aspden views the lumbar spine as an arch-like structure based on the anatomy of the muscles and ligaments and the stabilizing effects of intra-abdominal pressure and the thoracolumbar fascia during various lifting maneuvers.[24]

LATISSIMUS DORSI

The latissimus dorsi arises from the spinous processes of the lower six thoracic, the lumbar and the upper sacral vertebrae. In addition, it arises from the posterior part of the iliac crest and the lower four ribs via muscular slips that connect with slips of the origin of the external oblique. These fibers connect with the lumbodorsal fascia and a flattened tendon and insert into the crest of the lesser tubercle on the humerus. Because of its attachment to the lumbodorsal fascia, the latissimus dorsi is involved in generation of extensor moment and stabilization of the lumbar spine.[25]

The Thoracolumbar Fascia
or Lumbodorsal Fascia

Authorities differ on the structure and function of the thoracolumbar, or lumbodorsal fascia. Some believe the thoracolumbar fascia consists of three layers of fasciae that cover the muscles of the lumbar spine. Others believe that the true fascial layer is the anterior layer which consists of collagen fibers aligned in different directions. It covers the quadratus lumborum muscle. They believe that the other two layers are part of the aponeurosis since the collagen fibers are derived from the tendon of a muscle and are aligned in one direction.

According to Vleeming et al., the posterior layer of the fascia has multiple insertions, hence muscle-induced tension of this fascia assists in transferring loads between the spine, the pelvis, the legs and the arms.[26]

In addition to stabilizing the lower lumbar spine and the S1 joint, these authors maintain that this posterior layer of the thoracolumbar fascia aids in rotation of the trunk. Contraction of the gluteus medius and the powerful latissimus dorsi helps transfer forces to the posterior layer.

An understanding of the function and anatomy of the thoracolumbar fascia is essential to the appropriate design of techniques to relieve low back pain. Vleeming et al. argues that because the erector muscle is between the lateral raphe and the interspinous ligament, the deep lamina encloses it, and contraction of the muscle increases tension in the thoracolumbar fascia. Therefore, strengthening the erector spinae, gluteus and latissimus dorsi muscles strengthens the posterior layer of this fascia and increases closure force.[27]

Regarding the S1 joint, these authors point out that the biceps femoris and the gluteus maximus muscles are both attached to the sacrotuberous ligament which bridges the S1 joint and the contraction of these muscles aids in the transfer of loads across the joint. Pain around the S1 joint could be due to insufficient muscle action and resulting ligament strain.[27] This could be one of the reasons for S1 joint pain.

The role of sacroiliac joints in low back pain is intensely controversial, except in the specific instance of spondyloarthropathies.[28] Some point out that due to the complex topography of the joint it is virtually impossible for motions other than minor translations to take place. According to these authors a recent study found that there were no differences in motion in the painful sacroiliac joints with those patients with asymptomatic joints.[28] They concluded the weight of scientific evidence supports the concept that there is a limited role of the sacroiliac joints in low back pain except in the case of spondyloarthropathies. Nachemson writes "with regard to the sacroiliac pain syndromes, certain tests have been commonly used and results have indicated poor interrater reliability to the point that most authors agree that it is not possible to diagnose this syndrome. This finding has also been reinforced by the measurements of movements of these 'joints' by the roentgen stereophotogrammetric method."[29]

The only time S1 joint pain is seen and well-established in patients is associated with major trauma and the hormonal changes seen at pregnancy. However "pain in the sacroiliac and or pubic region of the pelvis has been alluded to as pelvic instability, and this is not a well documented pathologic entity. The validity of pelvic instability as a cause of low back pain and leg pain is the challenging issue."[30] Yet researchers like Julie Fritz[31] continue to study problems of the S1 joint with tests that are not valid and come to conclusions which are both erroneous and detrimental to patient care.

In my nearly 45 years of practice on three continents at major teaching hospitals, and later in private practice where I devoted all my time to the treatment of low back pain patients, I have not come across more than a handful of patients with this syndrome, and they were either due to major trauma or pregnancy.

Lumbodorsal fascia, according to McGill and others, is not a significant extensor of the spine, but a well-developed tissue with collagen fiber that probably acts as a natural extensor-muscle retinaculum, or abdominal corset around the lumbar spine to stabilize it. This corset is well innervated by Ruffini and Pacinian corpuscles, hence has a proprioceptive function.[32]

Other authors believe the effect of the lumbodorsal fascia is trivial, no more than 3-6 Nm, while a torque of about 200 Nm is needed to handle a heavy lift.[33]

The fascia has the following muscle connections: the transverses abdominis and internal oblique muscles are posterior attached; the latissimus dorsi attach to upper regions of the fascia; the back of the fascia wraps around the multifidus pars lumborum groups of iliocostalis and longissimus muscles. See Figure 4.

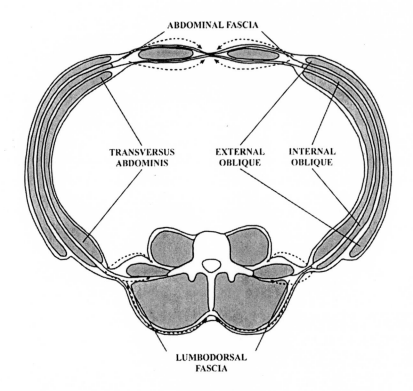

ABDOMINAL FASCIA

TRANSVERSUS ABDOMINIS

EXTERNAL OBLIQUE

INTERNAL OBLIQUE

LUMBODORSAL FASCIA

The abdominal fascia, anteriorly, and the LDF, posteriourly, are passive parts of the abdominal hoop. The lateral active musculature (transverse abdominis and internal oblique) serves to tension the hoop (dashed arrows).

Figure 4

THE MUSCLES OF THE ABDOMINAL WALL

The muscles of the abdominal wall can be divided into two

groups: (1) the medial muscles lying on either side of the midline, and (2) the lateral, the oblique (internal and external) muscles forming the anterolateral wall of the abdomen and ranging from superficial to deep: the external oblique, the internal oblique and the transversus abdominis which is the deep muscle.

The Medial Muscles of the Abdominal Wall

The **rectus abdomonis** on either side of the midline is enclosed by the aponeurosis of the **internal oblique muscle,** which splits into two fascial sheets that enclose the rectus abdomonis. The sheets criss-cross in the midline forming the *linea alba.* The four muscles are arrayed in distinctly different directions.

THE LATERAL MUSCLES OF THE TRUNK

The lateral muscles of the trunk are the quadratus lumborum and the psoas.

The Quadratus Lumborum

As its name implies, the quadratus lumborum is a quadrilateral sheet of muscle with attachments to the last rib, the iliac crest and the vertebral column. It is composed of three sets of fibers: (1) fibers from the last rib to the iliac crest, (2) fibers originating from the last rib and inserted into the transverse processes of the L5 vertebra, and (3) fibers originating from the first four lumbar vertebrae and inserted into the iliac crest.

The principle work of the quadratus is to brace the twelfth rib so that the lower thoracic fibers of the diaphragm can function.[34] When the quadratus acts on only one side along with the internal and external obliques, it flexes the trunk to that side.

Due to its architecture, the quadratus lumborum has a stabilizing effect on the lumbar spine under many loading actions, such as carrying weights in both hands. This is mainly due to its vertebral cross-link and large lateral-moment arm with the transverse processes.[35]

As an indication of its stabilizing function, the quadratus does not relax with the other extensors of the lumbar spine during the flexion-relaxation phenomenon.[36] The external oblique works in combination with the internal on the opposite side, thereby providing for rotation. The right external abdominal oblique, in concert with the left internal abdominal oblique, brings about rotation of the rib cage to the left. The rotation to the right has the reverse patterns of obliques. The obliques are important in low back health as the spine in the lumbar region is limited in rotation.

The Psoas Major

The psoas major is a unique muscle in that it crosses both the spine and the hip. Psoas major originates from the anterolateral aspect of the lumbar spine. At each level it arises from the transverse processes, from the intervertebral discs and adjacent margins, and finally from the tendinous arches covering the vertebral bodies. This long muscle then descends over the brim of the pelvis and inserts into the lesser trochanter of the femur.

It acts mainly to flex the thigh, but also in the reverse action, to flex the lumbar spine while the thigh is fixed. Nachemson considers the psoas major a major stabilizer of the lumbar spine.[37] But some investigators consider the psoas a lumbar stabilizer only in the presence of significant hip flexor torque.[38]

Studies by Parkkola et al.[39] have clearly demonstrated that two signs of muscle degeneration seen on MRI are decrease in muscle mass and fat deposits. In addition they noted that psoas and back muscles are smaller in old age, but only back muscles have fat deposits. This study also concluded that psoas and back muscles are smaller in patients with low back pain.

In patients with low back pain, the psoas muscle is weak.[40] For this reason, the senior author has long advocated eccentric exercises to strengthen the psoas muscle.[41] McGill urges caution when training this muscle because it's activation imposes a substantial compressive penalty on the spine.[42]

In 1968, a personal experience brought home the need for caution when working with the psoas muscle. While teaching a course at Rusk Rehab Center at NYU on the technique of training this muscle, I had my boss lying on the treatment table. I began to demonstrate on him the eccentric strengthening of the psoas. My second movement caused him severe pain, and only with much difficulty was he able, with my help, to rise from the treatment table! Ever since then, I have been extremely careful in using this technique on my patients.

THE LIGAMENTS

The spine is relatively flexible within its physiologic range of motion, but beyond this range, the ligaments resist forces and absorb large amounts of energy before failure occurs. When this bone-ligament-bone system is subjected to tensile loads, whether the bone or the ligament fails first depends on the rate of loading. When the rate of loading is slow, the bone fails first, and when the rate is high, the ligament fails first.[43] In practical terms, when one slips and falls, the high rate of loading can tear a ligament. And in sports, when injury occurs with the spine at the end of its range of motion, a ligament is apt to be torn.

Ligaments are bands of connective tissue that bind, or connect one bone or bony part to another. Most ligaments, made up of closely packed collagenous fibers, allow little stretching. But some, such as the ligament flava, consist of elastin fibers that stretch in one direction and rebound in the other, as a rubber band would.[43] In tension, the collagen fibers are stronger than the elastin fibers. Both are embedded in proteoglycan gel.

The ligaments are passive tissues, but it is important to realize that they undergo stress when the lumbar spine is engaged in flexion, extension or rotation movements, so they may be strained or sprained if loads surpass what the tissues can withstand.

Ligaments also have a proprioceptive function, as they are endowed with an extensive network of free nerve endings together with Ruffini corpuscles and Pacinian corpuscles.[44,45] The ligaments, as the primary restraints of the joints in the spinal column, play a significant role along with the muscles in stabilizing the lumbar spine. When the ligaments are subjected to various loads, the sensory receptors with which they are endowed elicit a reflex action in the paraspinal muscles, contributing to spinal stability. Solomonow et al.[46] speculate that their locations make the spinal ligaments sensitive to vertebral motions in various planes; their receptors monitor these movements, via spinal neurons, which activate the musculature to stabilize the spine.[46] They also surmise that the multifidus muscle, besides constantly providing stability to the spinal segments, which could be destabilized by heavy loads, also acts as a ligament whose tension is increased or decreased by neural control. Many other muscles may also be involved in stabilizing the spine, via ligamento-muscular reflexes. Even patients with disrupted posterior ligaments have few problems, because the reflex muscular activity from other ligaments or facet joints is enough to stabilize the spine. Solomonow et al.[46] conclude that muscle-strengthening therapy can not only improve spinal stability, but also prevent disabilities arising from breaks in stability that may occur from excessive load to muscles. Hence a sprain or tear of the ligament produces additional weakness.

In order to provide optimal therapy, the various roles of the spinal ligaments must be understood. These ligaments restrict motion within well-defined limits to protect the spinal cord. When heavy loads are suddenly applied, as in an automobile accident or a fall, the ligaments absorb the excessive amounts of energy, limiting displacement of the spinal structures to within safe limits.

Classification. The seven ligaments of the spine are classified into four groups, three of which are relevant to spinal stability and are discussed herein.

GROUP 1: The two ligaments that interconnect the vertebral bodies: the anterior longitudinal ligament and the posterior longitudinal ligament.

The anterior longitudinal ligament attaches to the anterior aspects of the vertebral bodies and discs. The attachment to the vertebral bodies is firm, but the attachment to the annular fibers of the discs is not as firm. Composed of collagen tissue, the ligament is directed longitudinally, hence resists vertical separation of the anterior ends of the vertebral bodies. During spinal extension, this ligament resists anterior bowing of the spine.

The posterior longitudinal ligament, as its name indicates, is posteriorly situated and covers the floor of the vertebral canal. This fibrous tissue is firmly attached to the edges of the vertebral bodies from the occiput to the sacrum. In the lumbar region, it forms a narrow band over the vertebral bodies but expands over the discs, giving it a serrated appearance. See Figures 5 and 6.

GROUP 2: The three ligaments that connect the posterior elements: the ligament flavum, the supraspinous ligament and the interspinous ligament.

The ligamentum flavum (Latin: flavus = yellow), known as

43

the yellow ligament, is made of large amounts of elastin fibers which are yellow in color when fresh. It connects the lower end of the internal aspect of one lamina to the upper end of the external surface of the lamina below. These ligaments tend to stretch when the spine bends forward. They shorten without buckling, which protects the neural elements; unless the ligamentum flavum loses elasticity from repeated injury.

The supraspinous ligament evidently is not a true ligament.[47] It consists of tendinous fibers of various muscles lying in the midline, and is attached to the posterior edges of the spinous processes of the lumbar spine. Its lower limit is the L5 spinous process. This structure resists forward bending of the intervertebral joints and prevents separation of the spinous processes.

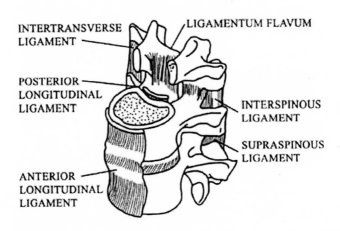

Ligaments of the spine. Besides the disc, there are seven ligaments that connect one vertebra to the next. Contribution to the spine stability by an individual ligament is dependent upon its cross-section, its distance from the instantaneous axis of rotation, and its orientation in space. The anatomy of the ligaments is such as to collectively provide stability to the spine in its various physiological motions.

Figure 5

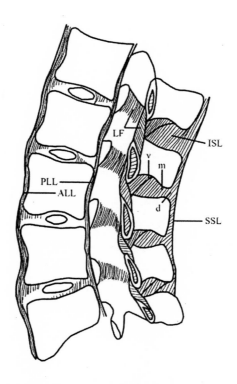

A median sagittal section of the lumbar spine to show its various ligaments: All – anterior longitudinal ligament. PLL – posterior longitudinal ligament. SSL – supraspinous ligament. ISL – interspinous ligament. V – ventral part; m – middle part; d – dorsal part. LF – ligamentum flavum, viewed from within the vertebral canal, and in sagittal section at the midline.

Figure 6

The interspinous ligament connects adjacent spinous processes and prevents their separation. The ligaments are thickest in the lumbar region where they limit flexion movements. Not all authorities agree regarding the orientation of its fibers. McGill[48] contends that they are oriented in an oblique direction. If this is true, it would explain the contraction-relaxation path of loading of the interspinous ligaments that may act to prevent vertebral displacement.

According to McGill, the interspinous ligament behaves like a collateral ligament, controlling vertebral rotation during flexion and helping the facet joint maintain contact while gliding. Its oblique orientation helps protect the ligament against posterior shear of the superior vertebra. Because of the oblique obliteration of its fibers, it is more apt to be injured by traumatic events than by lifting movements.[48]

GROUP 3: The ilio-lumbar ligament is the strongest ligament attached to the lumbar vertebral column. Its fibers originate at the tip and at the borders of the transverse process of L5 and pass backward and laterally to insert into the ilium. This ligament stabilizes the L5 vertebra, preventing it from rotating and sliding forward.

GROUP 4: These muscles are not directly involved in spinal stability.

SPINAL FORCES INVOLVED IN HEAVY LIFTING

Two contending theories have been advanced to account for the forces necessary to effect a heavy lifting motion of the spine: (1) intra-abdominal pressure theory, and (2) posterior ligamentous mechanism theory.

Intra-abdominal pressure theory postulates that intra-abdominal pressure exerts a compressive stress on the convex surface of the lumbar lordosis and this stress stiffens the lumbar spine.[49] This is particularly apparent in heavy weight-lifting; weight lifters are able to lift heavier weights when they maintain a lumbar lordosis than when they allow the lordosis to straighten or reverse.[50] The rise and fall of intra-abdominal pressure at the start of a lifting maneuver indicates that its stabilizing effect is greatest when it is most needed, such as when the load is being accelerated.[51] The thoracolumbar fascia restrains any radial extension of the back muscles, increasing their strength and stiffness. And the attachment of the fascia to the abdominal muscles synchronizes their stressing with the rise in intra-abdominal pressure so that together they stiffen the lumbar spine during bending and lifting.[51]

Cholwicki et al.[52] demonstrated that muscle stiffness is directly proportional to muscle force. In their study of a simplified model of the North American man, with respect to the L5-S1 joint, the trunk flexor force was 1550 N and the trunk extensor force was 2850 N. They concluded that in healthy persons, coactivation of the trunk flexor-extensor muscles provides mechanical stability to the lumbar spine in neutral postures.[52] They showed that in cases of injury entailing loss of spinal stiffness, muscle activity increases. This senior author, too, based on studies of muscle activity using surface EMG, has suggested this possibility and presented papers to that effect at various seminars. For patients with sciatic scoliosis due to disc herniation, the back extensors increase their activity in flexion, without the usual rest during the flexion-relaxation response. This results in the familiar levo-scoliotic posture contralateral to side of pain.

Interestingly, most individuals in the study of Cholwicki et al. exhibited an overlap of activity of flexor and extensor muscles. However, most maintained a constant level of activity of the internal oblique and multifidus muscles.[52] To sum up, we again emphasize the importance of strengthening all of the flexor and extensor muscles of the lumbar spine for someone with low back pain or injury.

Posterior ligamentous mechanism theory maintains that the muscles of the lumbar spine are not strong enough to aid in lifting actions using the spine as a lever. To perform such actions, the muscle power of the hip extensors must be transmitted via the lumbar spine to the trunk muscles and the upper limbs. But the extensors cannot do it alone either; they must be helped by the interspinous and supraspinous ligaments, the thoracolumbar fascia and the capsules of the facet joints. Gracovetsky et al. believe that during lifting, the abdominal muscles help flex the lumbar spine, and intra-abdominal pressure is a side effect having no direct bearing on the lifting.[53] This theory, although persuasive, has yet to be experimentally validated.

CHAPTER 3 NOTES

1. Moshe S. Ligamento-muscular stabilizing system of the spine. *Spine.* 1998; 23: 2552-2562.
2. White AA, Punjabi *MM. Clinical Biomechanics of the Spine.* 2nd ed. Philadelphia: Lippincott-Raven; 1990.
3. Moshe S. Ligamento-muscular stabilizing system of the spine. *Spine.* 23: 2552-2562.
4. Moshe S. Ligamento-muscular stabilizing system of the spine. *Spine.* 23: 2557.
5. Fernando CK. Treatment of low back pain. Proceedings of the world confederation for physical therapy. *7th International Congress;* 1974: 305-314.
6. Weinstein, S, Herring S. *The Spine in Sports.* New York: Orthopedic Update; 2002. T. Weinstein S, Herring S. *The Spine in Sports.* New York: Orthopedic Update; 2002.
7. Morris JM. Role of the trunk in the stability of the spine. *Journal of Bone and Joint Surgery.* 1961; 43A: No. 3.
8. Fernando CK. Treatment of low back pain. *Proceedings of the World Confederation for Physical Therapy'. 7th International Congress;* 1974: 305-314.
9. Eie N. Load capacity of the low back. *Journal of Oslo City Hospitals.* 1966; 16: 75-98.
10. Fernando CK. Establishing a ratio between Trunk Extensors and Flexors. Unpublished Study; 1968.
11. Bogduk N, Twomey LT. *Clinical Anatomy of the Lumbar Spine.* New York: Churchill Livingstone; 1987.
12. Adams M, Bogduk N, Burton K, Dolan P. *The Biomechanics*

of Back Pain Edinburgh: Churchill Livingstone; 2002: 32

13. Macintosh JE. The Bio-mechanics of the lumbar multifidus. *Clinical Biomechanics.* 1986; 1: 205-213.

14. Chowlewick, J. Lumbar spine stability can be augmented with an abdominal belt and/or increased intra-abdominal pressure. *European Spine Journal,* 8, 388-395.

15. Stokes I, et al. Selective changes in mutifidus dimensions in patients with chronic low back pain. In: Ulrich Q et al. Importance of the intersegmental trunk muscles for stability of the lumbar spine. *Spine.* 1998; 23: 1937-1945.

16. Pope, MH et al. Biomechanical definitions of spinal instability. *Spine.* 1985; 10: 255-256.

17. Stokes I, et al. Segmental motion and instability. *Spine.* 1987; 12: 688-691.

18. Bogduk N, et al. The universal model of the lumbar back muscles in the upright position. *Spine.* 1992; 17: 897-913.

19. Adams M, Bogduk N, Burton K, Dolan P. *The Biomechanics of Back Pain* Edinburgh: Churchill Livingstone; 2002: 42.

20. McGill S. *Low Back Disorders.* Champaign, IL: Human Kinetics; 2002; 67.

21. Fernando CK, Samo JE. Low back pain: A new rationale and technique of treatment by therapeutic exercises. *Proceedings of the First International Assembly.* Asian Pacific League of Physical Medicine; 1970: 106-109.

22. McGill S. *Law Back Disorders.* Champaign, IL: Human Kinetics; 2002: 67.

23. Aspden RM. Review of the functional anatomy of the spinal ligaments and the lumbar erector spinae muscles. *Clinical Anatomy.* 1992; 2 '.372-387.

24. McGill S. *Low Back Disorders.* Champaign, IL: Human Kinetics; 2002: 68.

25. Vieeming A. The posterior layers of the Thoracolumbar

Fascia: Its function in load transfer from spine to legs. *Spine.* 1995; 7: 753-758

26. Vleeming A. The posterior layers of the Thoracolumbar Fascia: Its function in load transfer from spine to legs. *Spine.* 1995; 7: 757.

27. Frymoyer JW, Gordon SL. *New Perspectives on Low Back Pain.* Park Ridge, SL: American Academy of Orthopedic Surgeons; 1989: 241.

28. Nachemson A. *Neck and Back Pain.* Philadelphia: Lippincott; 2000: 195.

29. White AA, Punjabi *MM.. Clinical Biomechanics of the Spine.* 2nd ed. Philadelphia: Lippincott-Raven; 1990: 61.

30. Fritz JM, et al. Factors related to the inability of individuals with low back pain to improve with a spinal manipulation. *Physical Therapy.* 2004; 84: 173-190

31. Yahia LH, Newman N. Neurohistory of the lumbar spine. *Acta Orth Scand.* 1998; 59: 508-512.

32. Macintosh JE, Bogduk N. Biomechanics of the thoracolumbar fascia. *Clinical'Biomechanics.* 1987; 2: 78-83.

33. Adams M, Bogduk N, Burton K, Dolan P. *The Biomechanics of Back Pain.* Edinburgh: Churchill Livingstone; 2002: 33.

34. McGill S. *Law Back Disorders.* Champaign, IL: Human Kinetics; 2002: 74.

35. Andersen, et al. EMG activities of the quadrates lumborum and erector spinae muscles during flexion-relaxation and other motor tasks. *Clinical Biomechanics.* 1996; 11: 392-400.

36. Nachemson A. Possible importance of the psoas muscle for the lumbar spine. *Acta Ortha Scand.* 1968; 39: 47-57.

37. McGill S. *Low Back Disorders.* Champaign, IL: Human Kinetics; 2002: 73.

38. Parkkola, et al. MRI trunk muscle and psoas. *Spine.* 1993; 18:

830-833.

39. Alston W. Quantitative study of muscle factors in the chronic low back syndromes. *Journal of the American Geriatric Society.* 1966; 14: 1041-1047.

40. Fernando CK, Samo JE. Low back pain: A new rationale and technique of treatment by therapeutic exercises. *Proceedings of the First International Assembly.* Asian Pacific League of Physical Medicine; 1970: 106-109.

41. McGill S. *Low Back Disorders.* Champaign, IL: Human Kinetics; 2002: 74.

42. White AA, Punjabi MM. *Clinical Biomechanics of the Spine.* 2nd ed. Philadelphia: Lippincott- Raven; 1990: 19-28.

43. Jiang HJ. Nature and distribution of the innervation of human supraspinal and intestinal ligaments. *Spine.* 1995; 20: 869-876.

44. Solmonow M. Ligamento-muscular stabilization system of the spine. *Spine.* 1998; 23: 2552-2562.

45. Solmonow M. Ligamento-muscular stabilization system of the spine. *Spine.* 1998; 23: 2553.

46. Adams M, Bogduk N, Burton K, Dolan P. *The Biomechanics of Back Pain.* Edinburgh: Churchill Livingstone; 2002: 21.

47. McGill S. *Low Back Disorders.* Champaign, IL: Human Kinetics; 2002: 77.

48. Aspden R. Review of the functional anatomy of the spinal ligaments and the lumbar erector spinae muscles. *Clinical Anatomy.* 1992; 5: 373.

49. Porter RW. *Management of Back Pain.* Edinburgh: Churchill Livingstone; 1986.

50. Aspden, R. Review of the functional anatomy of the spinal ligaments and the lumbar erector spinae muscles. *Clinical Anatomy.* 1992; 5: 372-387.

51. Cholwicki J. Stabilizing function of trunk flexor-extensor

muscles around a neutral spine posture. *Spine.* 1997; 22: 2207-2212.

52. Gracovetsky S. Abdominal mechanism. *Spine.* 1985; 10: 317-324.

IV

JOINTS OF THE LUMBAR SPINE

The basic segment of the spine involved in movement is a three-joint complex consisting of one interbody joint, which is the intervertebral disc between the bodies of adjacent vertebrae, also known as the fibrocartilaginous joint, and two synovial joints, which are the zygapophysial, or facet joints between the articular processes of adjacent vertebrae.[1] Stability of this three-joint complex depends on the integrity of the intervertebral disc.

Thus, the articulations of the lumbar spine are three: (1) between two adjacent vertebral bodies, the interposed fibro-cartilaginous disc — a strong joint, strengthened anteriorly and posteriorly by anterior and posterior longitudinal ligaments; and (2 & 3) the two synovial joints between the articular processes of adjacent vertebrae — the zygapophysial, or facet joints.

Some fusion between the L5 vertebra and the sacrum, known as sacralization is present in about 5.5% of the population in the U.S. An elongated thoracolumbar segment, due to partial or complete separation of the first sacral vertebra from the sacrum, known as lumbarization, is present in about 6% of people in the U.S. When a sacralization or lumbarization is present unilaterally, the articulations at that level are asymmetrical, tending to dispose the individual to back problems.

MOVEMENTS OF THE VERTEBRAL COLUMN

The discs and the facet joints enable the bodies of the vertebrae to move upon each other, which allows movement of the entire vertebral column. Other factors check the motion of these joints, namely, the ratio of the height of the disc to the height of the bony part of the vertebra, and the ligaments and the muscles.

The interbody joints allow for the majority of motions: flexion and extension in the sagittal plane, lateral flexion in the horizontal plane and axial rotation. The synovial joints limit the range of movement between any two vertebrae, thus the movement of the vertebral column as a whole ultimately depends on the orientation of the articular facet joints.

In the lumbar region, the discs are thick and the vertical articular surfaces are sagittally oriented. This allows relatively free flexion and extension, with minimal lateral flexion and limited rotation, due to the shape and orientation of the articular processes, which oppose each other in a sagittal plane. The facets of the last two lumbar vertebrae, however, are oriented in the frontal plane, allowing more rotation here.

MOBILITY AND STABILITY

Mobility and stability are important attributes of the vertebral column. Mobility of the vertebral column is mainly due to the elasticity and compressibility of the intervertebral discs. The muscles, joints and ligaments also play important roles. Stability depends on the normal curves of the spine and the strength of the vertebral bodies, joints, ligaments and muscles. In addition, stability of the spine depends on its articulations. Abnormal articulations or narrowing of the intervertebral discs due to degeneration, herniation or abnormal posture can strain the facet joints and the posterior ligaments, causing pain and instability.

POSTURE

Posture, it must be remembered, is controlled involuntarily. When the influence of gravity disturbs it, posture is normally corrected involuntarily.[2] Any movement of the trunk, head or arms can shift the center of gravity so as to provoke muscle activity that could lead to muscle fatigue and pain if prolonged.

In normal posture, a plumb line from the earlobe falls through the center of the shoulders, through the center of the hip and toward the front of the knee, ending in front of the lateral malleolus. The head is erect and well-balanced with the chin in. Ideally, the vertebral curves are such that action in the muscles is minimal (see figure 7). In about 75% of individuals the line of gravity passes in front of the mid-L4 vertebra; gravity tends to pull the lumbar spine and thorax into flexion. To oppose this, the posterior muscles of the back, chiefly the multifidus and the sagittal rotators, are constantly active. The opposite is true when the line of gravity passes behind the lumbar spine; in this case, gravity tends to pull the lumbar spine and thorax into extension.[3]

In ideal normal posture, adjacent vertebrae rest upon each other with no problems. Several situations, however, generate high stress on normal, undamaged spinal structures. For instance, adjacent vertebrae pressing on each other at an unusual angle concentrate a high amount of stress on intervertebral discs, ligaments and facet joints. Another problematic situation is sustained loading of the intervertebral discs, which can cause loss of water in the disc and consequent loss of disc height, known as viscoelastic creep.[4] This loss can reduce the capacity of discs to equalize stress. A third stressful situation occurs when muscles are disproportionately activated. This adversely affects normal spinal mechanics and so reduces the muscles normal protection of the spine.

A lordotic spine (Figure 7) is associated with a posteriorly bulging disc and also with greater intradiscal pressure.[5] Good abdominal musculature is therapeutic and maintains correct posture, which considerably reduces both the bulge and the pressure on the posterior disc.[5]

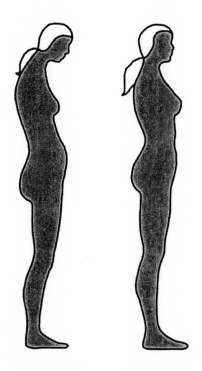

The posture of patients with a lordotic spine (left) is associated with posterior bulging of the disc and also with greater intradiscal pressure. Both factors are reduced considerably by correct posture (right), which is maintained by good abdominal musculature, also of therapeutic value.

Figure 7

Various pathological-anatomical factors which have been described can cause poor posture. The simplistic view that muscles are responsible for postural deviations is incorrect. But Braggins and others reported by Braggins, such as Commerford, who accept the view that stretching shortened muscles and strengthening weakened muscles in a corrective and reeducation program[6] are promoting exercises in futility.

Interactions of the Interbody Joint and the Facet Joints

At the same time that the major movements of the interbody joint described previously take place in the three principal planes, several other motions simultaneously take place in the sagittal plane. In lumbar flexion, anterior translation and rotation occur, and in lumbar extension, posterior translation and rotation occur. Translation and rotation take place within the five vertebrae of the lumbar spine.[7]

Translation is forward or backward sliding of the vertebrae due to sheer force of gravity and muscle action. The anatomical design of the lumbar intervertebral joints makes them resistant to anterior translation.

Rotation is twisting of the interbody joint and the facet joints in the horizontal plane.

The interbody joint and the facet (zygapophysial) joints work together to bring about movement. The interbody joint by itself could move unrestrictedly in all directions if the posterior elements of the vertebra were removed. Thus the operation of the interbody joint cannot be described without discussing the operation of the facet joints as well.

Movement of the interbody is possible in all directions; the vertebrae can press together in weight-bearing, or they can be distracted, or separated, which is relevant during treatment (traction or distraction). The interbody can slide forward, backward or sideways; it can also rock forward, backward or sideways.[8] Frequently these compound motions of the vertebral body and disc complex are involved in bending, and reaching and lifting actions.

The facet (zygapophysial) joint, a typical synovial joint is composed of the inferior articular process of one vertebra with the superior articular process of the vertebra above it. The articular facet is lined with hyaline cartilage and the whole structure is contained in an articular capsule composed of an inner synovial membrane and outer fibrous membrane. Meniscoids of a fibroadipose substance form around the facet rims. Their alleged involvement in lock-back syndrome has yet to be proven. According to Kos and Wolf, meniscoids can become trapped in the lumbar facet joints, causing locked back; this theory is advocated by proponents of treatment by manipulation.[9] But Bogduk et al. dismiss this theory as unsound because in the flexed position, the articular facets are subluxated, so the meniscoid structures are drawn out of the joint cavity.[10] See Figure 8.

The synovial joints lie posterior to the emerging nerves so that any undue inflammation of the joint can irritate these nerves and cause pain. Blockage of venous drainage in the intervertebral foramen will compromise the root and/or dorsal root ganglion at that level.[11]

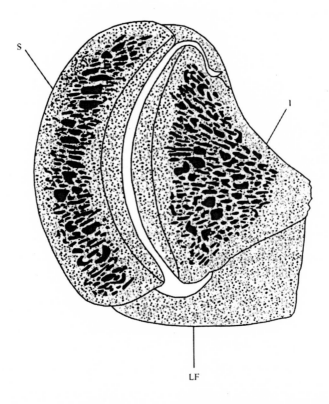

A transverse (horizontal) section through a lumbar zygapophysial joint. Note how the posterior capsule is fibrous and attaches to the inferior articular pricess (I) well beyond the articular margin, but at its other end it attaches to the superior articular process (S) and the margin of the articular cartilage. The anterior capsule is formed by the ligamentum flavum (LF).

Figure 8

The shape and plane of the articular surfaces determine the range of movement of the synovial joints in the lumbar region. The first three joints in this region are more sagittally oriented than are the fourth and fifth, which are oriented in a frontal plane. In the upper lumbar region, facets of the superior articular processes largely face laterally while those of the inferior articular processes largely face medially. The thickness of the discs and the sagittal position of the synovial joints in the upper three lumbar vertebrae allow the large range of flexion, extension and lateral flexion movements in this area. At the same time, only minimal rotation is possible because the articular surfaces lock almost immediately. In the fourth and fifth vertebrae, however, the lower facets are oriented frontally, so more rotation can take place at these levels. As Figure 9 shows, the articular surfaces are vertical in the upper lumbar spine and more oblique in the lower lumbar area. See Figure 9.

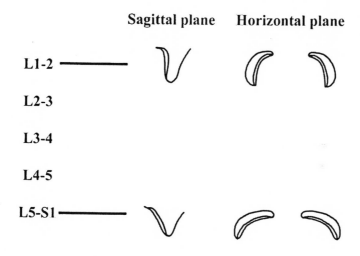

The orientation of the zygapophysial joints varies with lumbar level, in both the sagittal and horizontal planes. Changes are gradual between L1-L2 and L5-S1. Cartilage-covered articular surfaces are shown hatched.

Figure 9

61

This vertical orientation of the facet joints in the lumbar region permits flexion and extension and limiting side flexion and rotation. These previous factors limit the stress to the annular fibers of the disc. The opposition of the articular surfaces of the facet joints, the joint capsule and the posterior ligament provides resistance, limiting the range of flexion.[12] The inferior joint facet, which opposes the lamina of the vertebra below it, limits extension, and the spinous processes, which impact on each other, limit extreme extension. If the spine is thrown into hyperextension, as in vehicular accidents or sports injuries, the interspinous ligament is ruptured or torn."

Of the three joints, the interbody joint and the two facet joints, the interbody joint bears the most weight and is responsible for nearly 80% of the weight-bearing compressive load. The facet joints play a substantial role in stabilization, however, as do the normal curves of the spine and the integrity of the vertebrae and the ligaments binding them together.[14] The Wedge Maneuver, performed on patients with scoliotic list, an indication of an early disc lesion, must also be mentioned. Proponents of the McKenzie protocols also call the maneuver "slide gliding," a misnomer because no such movement can take place in the three-joint complex. Another name, "pelvic translocation," has replaced earlier used names, "lateral shift" and "lateral gliding." All are misnomers. Such motions do not and cannot take place in the interbody joint. According to Fritz, "pelvic translocation" describes the movement in which the pelvis is shifted relative to the shoulders in the frontal plane.[15] Why Woodman spends time on study and research of a maneuver that cannot take place is beyond comprehension.[16]

RANGE OF MOTION OF THE LUMBAR SPINE

Range of motion of the spine varies with age, gender and time of day. During the day, fluid is expelled from the discs, which increases the range of flexion of the lumbar spine by 5 to 6.5 degrees in healthy subjects and 11 degrees in patients with back pain.[17] The range of lateral bending also increases.[17] The range of extension, however, is unaffected.[17]

Also, it must be remembered that in normal, healthy adults, a vigorous training program can increase the range of flexion by 5 degrees and lateral bending by 9 degrees. But the same process seems incapable of increasing the range of extension.[17]

As mentioned, the normal movements of the lumbar spine are flexion and extension in the sagittal plane, lateral flexion in the coronal plane, and axial rotation in the horizontal plane. Two additional movements are biomechanically incorporated, namely axial compression and axial distraction.

In flexion/extension, the range of motion increases from the LI to L5/S1 level. The L5/S1 joint allows more movement in flexion/extension than do the other lumbar joints. In lateral flexion and axial rotation, however, the L5/S1 joint allows less motion than do the other lumbar joints.

The last two vertebral joints, namely L4/L5 and L5/S1, are more susceptible to disc disease than the other lumbar vertebral joints, possibly because these two joints have a greater range of movement in the sagittal plane and are exposed to greater weight-bearing than the other joints of the lumbar spine.

One of the principle functions of the facet joints is to maintain the stability of the lumbar spine in flexion. When the lumbar spine flexes forward, the vertebrae slide forward due to a combination of gravity and muscle action, in a motion called translation. The articular surfaces of the facet joints then impact on each other, arresting this action and maintaining stability. The amount of translation, then, is a measure of the stability or instability of the lumbar spine. According to Pearcy, 2 mm of translation in the lumbar spine is normal.[18] After careful study of all factors, White & Punjabi agree that 4.5mm of translation indicates instability.[19]

Many structures are involved in resisting flexion in the lumbar spine. According to Adams et al., the intervertebral disc contributes about 29%, supraspinous and interspinous ligaments about 19%, yellow elastic ligament (ligamentum flavum) about 19%, and the facet joint capsule about 39%. These structures limit flexion only in the sagittal plane.[20]

Flexion motions of the normal lumbar spine as averaged by White & Punjabi range as follows[21] (in degrees):

Gross flexion	56
L1/L2	8
L2/L3	10
L3/L4	12
L4/L5	13
L5/S1	9

Extension motions of the normal lumbar spine, as averaged by Pearcy et al, and Pearcy & Tibrewal, range as follows [22, 23] (in degrees):

L1/L2	5
L2/L3	3
L3/L4	1
L4/L5	2
L5/S1	5

During flexion and extension, translation and rotation occur at each segment. Lumbar flexion involves anterior translation and rotation, while extension involves posterior translation and rotation in the sagittal plane, as mentioned.

Extension movements are stabilized by the anterior longitudinal ligament, the facet joints and the anterior aspect of the annulus fibrosus.[24-25] Extension of the basic segments involved in lumbar movement is limited when the inferior articular surface of the facet impacts on the lamina of the vertebra below, thereby blocking farther motion. When the force on the facet joints is extreme, the capsule may rupture; this could then cause back pain on extension.[26]

Lateral Flexion

Lateral flexion of the lumbar spine is a complex movement taking place in both the interbody joints and the facet joints. Clinical studies of these movements have as yet produced no definite conclusions, however, the limitations seen in lateral flexion and other movements of the lumbar spine aid our understanding of the aging process and/or degeneration of the segments involved.

The range of lateral flexion movements decreases with age, according to radiographic measurements and studies of living subjects and cadavers. Range average as follows [27, 28]:

	Degrees	Left	Right
Gross Lateral Flexion		18	25
L1/L2		5	6
L2/L3		5	6
L3/L4		5	6
L4/L5		3	5
L5/S1		0	2

Axial Rotation

Axial rotation, the twisting that takes place in the horizontal plane, involves both the interbody joint and the facet joints. The annulus resists the movement; half the collagen fibers of the annulus stretch and the other half are relaxed. This strains the lamellae of the annulus and if the highly innervated three or four outer layers are strained, this can cause pain. The range of axial rotation averages as follows[27, 28]:

	Degrees	Left	Right
Gross Axial Rotation		5	6
L1/L2		1	1
L2/L3		1	1
L3/L4		1	2
L4/L5		1	2
L5/S1		1	0

Rotation beyond 3 degrees injures the collagen fibers of the annulus.[29] The facet joints and the posterior ligaments protect the intervertebral disc from further injury. Studies of Farfan, reported by Bogduk and Twomey, clearly show that during axial rotation the disc contributes 35% of the resistance to torsion and the posterior elements, namely the facet joints, supraspinous and intraspinous ligaments, contribute 65%.[30]

Axial Compression

Axial compression is the movement that occurs during weight-bearing in the upright postition.[31] In this axial compression, the components of the intervertebral disc, mainly the nucleus pulposus and the annulus, transmit the weight downward from one vertebra to another. The weight is transmitted via the end plates and it is believed that the end plates fracture before any other structure during weight-bearing. The central part of the end plate fractures first according to Horst[32], indicating that the part over the nucleus pulposus is weaker than the part over the annulus.

The facet joints certainly do not bear much weight on compression and it is now believed that all the weight is borne by the interbody joints.[33] Adams et al. showed that when the disc is narrowed due to disease, nearly 70% of axial loading is carried by the inferior articular processes of the facet joints and lamina. In prolonged standing, subjects with a lordotic spine have impacted facet joints; L3/L4, L4/L5 and L5/S1 bear 19% of the load while the upper joints bear only 11%. Thus lordosis enables a person to bear additional axial compression.[33]

Creep

Under constant loading, the disc loses fluid and this process, known as creep, is responsible for the changes in an individual's height from day to night. After a 16 hour day performing the various activities of daily life — walking, sitting and standing — 20% of disc height is lost, resulting in the individual being 15-25 mm shorter.[34] Tyrell et al. showed that the return to full disc height is more rapid if one flexes the lower limbs instead of lying supine in an extended position. This flexed position is used in therapy for back pain.[35]

Axial Distraction

Distraction, or pulling apart, is not a normal movement of the lumbar spine. The drawing apart of the vertebrae is a treatment called traction, used for disc lesions. One of the earliest users of this therapeutic technique was Cyriax.[36]

Traction: 1) increases the separation between vertebrae so that loose fragments can move, 2) eases pain so the patient can relax, 3) tightens the posterior longitudinal ligament to create a centripetal force and 4) produces suction, adding further centripetal force and 5) disconnects the facet joints.[36] According to Cyriax, sustained traction is like enhanced bed rest: it not only eliminates compression, it decompresses.[36]

Traction not only eases back pain due to disc herniations, it also produces negative intradiscal pressure which has a therapeutic effect on the disease process.[37] The decompression tensions used in these studies, from 50 to 100 lbs, significantly reduced the intradiscal pressures to minus 150-160 mm Hg.

To be effective, traction must be sustained. After two minutes, the muscles tire and relax so that the distracting force then acts on the ligaments. Intermittent traction is self-defeating because it does not allow the muscles time to relax.

At least 40-90 kg of traction is needed to be effective for the lumbar region.[37] The amount of traction used in hospitals, 7-9 kg of traction with a pelvic harness, is insufficient and has no effect on disc lesions, its only value being to quiet the patient.

Twomey performed a study where he applied 9 kg of traction to lumbar spines of cadavers.[38] Since physical therapists apply much higher weights on patients, this study is of not clinical significance.

THE LUMBOSACRAL JUNCTION

The vertebral column curves markedly at the cervicothoracic, thorocolumbar and lumbosacral junctions, allowing increased mobility at these sites. For this reason, these sites are more susceptible to damage and disease than other parts of the spine. Indeed, vertebral fractures are more common at these sites than elsewhere.

Of the three curves, the lumbosacral junction takes the sharpest change in direction and bears the greatest weight as well. The shapes of both the discs and the vertebrae in this region account for the radical shape of the curve. In the upper part of the curve, the discs are wedge-shaped and thicker anteriorly than posteriorly. Lower down, disc is similarly shaped and the L5 vertebrae is also thicker anteriorly than posteriorly, further intensifying the curvature.

When standing upright, the sacrum inclines downward nearly 30-50 degrees from the horizontal. This can cause the L5 vertebrae to slip on the sacrum, but ordinarily this does not happen. The reason it does not happen is believed to be that the inferior articular processes of the L5 vertebrae snugly engage the sacrum, preventing the slippage. Another reason is that the strength of the ligaments, mainly the iliolumbar ligaments, strongly secures the L5 transverse processes to the ilium on each side. Finally, according to Adams & Bogduk the auricular surface of the lateral area of the sacrum locks onto a roughened ligamentous surface behind the auricular surface, helping to keep the sacrum inside the pelvic rim and prevent forward slippage.[39]

The lumbosacral joint allows more motion in the sagittal plane than do the other lumbar joints, as studies by Lumsden et al. demonstrate.[40] In lateral bending and in axial rotation, however, the lumbosacral joint allows less motion than do the other lumbar joints.[40] The hypothesis seems reasonable, then, that the L4/L5 and L5/S1 joints, since they carry more weight and have a wider range of movement in the sagittal plane, may be more susceptible to disease than the other joints.

COUPLED MOTIONS

Unintended motions sometimes take place in one joint at the same time as an intentional movement in another joint. Studies by Pearcy and Tibrewal demonstrate that flexion of lumbar intervertebral joints are coupled with rotation, translation and a few degrees of axial and coronal rotations.[41] Extension movements involve sagittal rotation and posterior translation. Pearcy and Tribrewal give details of coupled movements with lateral flexion and axial rotation as well.[41] Because of its anatomical design, the lumbar intervertebral disc is resistant to anterior translation, and its movement is parallel to the body due to shear force. It is also thought to resist axial rotation. At the same time, it allows sagittal and frontal plane rotations.[43] Increased coupled motions are associated with narrowing of disc space, according to clinical studies. Axial rotations greater than 4 degrees coupled with extension or flexion are abnormal and cause for alarm according to Pearcy et al.[44]

Men have more mobility in the sagittal plane than women. Women have a greater range of lateral flexion than men. Many studies indicate that with age, both men and women lose mobility in sagittal and frontal planes. This senior author agrees that mobility decreases in all planes due to low back problems, because movement exacerbates any pain. Decreased mobility, however, cannot serve as a diagnostic criterion to differentiate the cause of back pain.[45, 46, 47]

STABILITY

Clinical instability may develop in the lumbar spine due to disc degeneration, spinal stenosis, spondylolysis, spondylolisthesis, or a neurologic deficit due to a burst fracture. The instability may cause a bony fragment to be pushed into the neural canal. This can be managed in the lumbar area, unlike in the cervical or the thoracic, because: 1) There is available space in the lumbar spinal canal, 2) The large muscles around the lumbar spine — the abdominals, erector spinae, psoas and the quadratus lumborum — act as a corset to stabilize the lumbar spine.[48, 49] Any injury to the cauda-equina is a problem of the lower motor neuron, which regenerates so that complete muscle function returns. On the other hand, an injury to the cervical or thoracic spinal cord is a problem of the upper motor neuron and the end result is less return of function.

Many authorities believe that the causes of low back pain are not well understood. Some believe that depression and poor job satisfaction are related to low back pain. Others believe mechanical disorders cause spinal instability.[50] White and Punjabi propose a checklist for clinical instability of the lumbar spine where points are assigned to various damaged structures and five or more points indicates clinical instability.[51]

Studies of the spinal stabilizing system began with Knutson's use of radiography.[52] Since then, it has been demonstrated that an isolated ligamentous spine fixed at its base will collapse under a force of only 4 and 1/2 pounds.

The new studies of Punjabi[53] are an important improvement on the old theories; he speaks of three subsystems that subserve the spinal stabilizing system: 1. Spinal column; 2. Spinal muscles surrounding the spinal column; 3. Motor-control unit. According to Punjabi, the three subsystems work together to provide spinal stability. He argues that any problem with any of the parts of this system will cause instability. It is thought that the spine is flexible at low loads and stiffens with increasing loads. This can be represented by a bowl and a ball. The shape of the bowl represents spinal stability; e.g. a deeper bowl like a wine glass is representative of a stable spine and a shallow bowl like a soup plate is representative of an unstable spine. It is explained that in the soup plate the ball moves easily and hence has a larger neutral zone than in the wine glass, as the ball cannot move up the slopes easily, and hence a smaller neutral zone. According to Punjabi, the neutral zone is part of the range of motion. According to McGill[54], stability involves "achieving the stiffness needed to endure unexpected loads preparing for moving quickly, and ensuring sufficient stiffness in any degree of freedom of the joint that may be compromised from injury." Motor control fitness is essential for achieving the stability target under all possible conditions for performance and injury avoidance.

THE MOTOR CONTROL UNIT

When Punjabi and McGill speak of a motor-control unit, it seems to me they are discussing a theoretical construct rather than an anatomical-pathological entity. Motor control is mediated on an involuntary basis rather than a voluntary basis. According to the anatomical understanding, motor-control is governed by two systems: the upper motor neurone and the lower motor neurone. When these two systems are injured due to disease or trauma, they exhibit certain characteristic features. Lower motor neurone lesions will show the following characteristic features: 1. paralysis of the muscles innervated by these fibers, 2. Loss of muscle tone, 3. Disuse atrophy of affected muscles, 4. Deep tendon reflexes diminished. This is seen in diseases affecting the anterior horn cells or injury to the ventral roots of peripheral nerves. In case of disease or injury to the upper motor neurone, the following characteristic features are seen: 1. Paresis or paralysis of the muscles, after some initial loss of muscle tone, followed by increase tonus of anti-gravity muscles, i.e. spasticity, 2. Hyperactive deep tendon reflexes, 3. Positive Babinski sign. The senior author wonders what happens in the case of injury to the motor-control unit! Finally it must be remembered that spinal instability is one sign or symptom of mechanical disorders of the lumbar spine. If patients are treated with diagnosis driven therapy then these signs and symptoms will be addressed in the treatment protocols. Some physical therapists[55] seem to compare protocols of knee joint instability with those with spinal instability, and lament studies have not been done with unstable surfaces like therapy balls for the treatment of these unstable back problems. The senior author's urgent plea is never to subject low back pain patients to treatment on unstable surfaces for the very fear that this might increase intradiscal pressures, which could cause greater harm than we are asked to solve. Finally, it must be remembered that due to the anatomical reasons mentioned earlier that spinal instability in the lumbar region is a lesser problem to treat than at the thoracic and cervical regions.

CHAPTER 4 NOTES

1. Bogduk N, Twomey L. *Clinical Anatomy of the Lumbar Spine.* Melbourne: Churchill Livingstone; 1987: 11-32.
2. Bogduk N, Twomey L. *Clinical Anatomy of the Lumbar Spine.* Melbourne: Churchill Livingstone; 1987: 86.
3. Assmussen E. Form and function of the erect human spine. *Clinic of Orthopedics.* 1962; 25: 55-63.
4. Kraemer J, Kolditz D, Gowin R. Water and electrolyte content of human intervertebral disc under variable load. *Spine.* 1985; 10: 69-71.
5. White A, Punjabi MM. *Clinical Biomechanics of the Spine.* 2nd ed. Philadelphia: Uppincott-Raven; 1990: 428.
6. Braggins, S. *Back Care: a Clinical Approach.* Edinburgh: Churchill Livingstone; 2000:153.
7. White AA, Punjabi *MM. Clinical Biomechanics of the Spine.* 2nd ed. Philadelphia: Lippincott-Raven; 1990: 86-125.
8. Bogduk N, Twomey L. *Clinical Anatomy of the Lumbar Spine.* Melbourne: Churchill Livingstone; 1987: 11-32.
9. Kos J, Wolf J. As reported in: Bogduk N, Twomey LT. *Clinical Anatomy of the Lumbar Spine.* Melbourne: Churchill Livingstone; 1987: 140.
10. Bogduk N, Twomey L. *Clinical Anatomy of the Lumbar Spine.* Melbourne: Churchill Livingstone; 1987: 140.
11. Twomey LT, Taylor JR. *Physical Therapy of the Low Back.* New York: Churchill Livingstone; 2000.
12. Adams M, Hutton WC, Stott JR. The resistance to flexion of the lumbar intervertebral joint. *Spine.* 1980; 5: 245-253.

13. Adams M, Bogduk N, Burton K, Dolan P. *Biomechanics of Back Pain.* Edinburgh: Churchill Livingstone; 2002:117.

14. Hollingshead WH. *Textbook of Anatomy.* 2nd ed. New York: Harper & Row; 1967: 321.

15. Fritz JM. Use of a classification approach in the treatment of three patients with low back *syndrome. American Physical Therapy Association.* 1998: 84-95.

16. Woodman R, Ralston P, Dufresne M. Reduction of a lumbar disc lesion using the wedge maneuver: a clinical report. *Physical Therapy.* 1985; 65: 346-350.

17. Ensink FB, Saur PM, Frese K, et al. Lumbar range of motion: influence of time and individual factors on measurements. *Spine.* 1996; 21:1339-1343.

18. Pearcy M, Portek I, Shephered J. Three dimensional X-ray analysis of normal movement of the lumbar spine. *Spine.* 1984; 9: 294-297.

19. White AA, Punjabi *MM.. Clinical Biomechanics of the Spine.* 2nd ed.. Philadelphia: Lippincott-Raven; 1990: 106.

20. Adams M. Resistance of flexion of the lumbar intervertebral joint. *Spine.* 1980; 5: 245-253.

21. White AA, Punjabi MM. *Clinical Biomechanics of the Spine.* 2nd ed. Philadelphia: Lippincott-Raven; 1990.

22. Pearcy M, Portek I, Shepherd J. Three dimensional X-ray analysis of normal movement of the lumbar spine. *Spine.* 1984; 9: 294-297.

23. Pearcy M, Tibrewal SB. Axial rotation and lateral bending in the normal lumbar spine measured by three dimensional radiography. *Spine.* 1984; 9: 582-587.

24. Haher TR, O'brien M, Dryer JW, Nucci R, Zipnick R, Leone DJ. Role of the lumbar facet joints in spinal stability. Identification of alternative paths of loading. *Spine.* 1994; 19: 2667-2670.

25. Sharma M, Langrana NA, Rodriguez J. Role of ligaments and facets in lumbar spine stability. *Spine.* 1995; 9: 887-900.

26. Yang KH, King AI. Mechanism of facet load transmission as a hypothesis for low back pain. *Spine.* 1984; 9: 557-565.

27. Pearcy M, Portek I, Shepherd J. Three dimensional X-ray analysis of normal movement of the lumbar spine. *Spine.* 1984; 9: 294-297.

28. Pearcy M, Tibrewal SB. Axial rotation and lateral bending in the normal lumbar spine measured by three dimensional radiography. *Spine.* 1984; 9: 582-587.

29. Hickey DS, Hurkin DWL. Relation between the structure of the annulus fibrosus and failure of the intervertebral disc. *Spine.* 1980; 5: 100-116.

30. Farfan HF, Cossette JW, Robertson GH, Wells RV, Kraus H. The effects of torsion on the lumbar intervertebral joints: The role of torsion in the production of disc degeneration, In Bogduk, N, Twomey L, Eds. *Clinical Anatomy of the Lumbar Spine.* Melbourne: Churchill Livingstone; 1970:67.

31. Farfan HF, Cossette JW, Robertson GH, Wells RV, Kraus H. The effects of torsion on the lumbar intervertebral joints: The role of torsion in the production of disc degeneration. In Bogduk N, Twomey L, Eds. *Clinical Anatomy of the Lumbar Spine.* Melbourne: Churchill Livingstone; 1970: 53.

32. Horst M. Measurement of the distribution of axial stress on the end plate of the vertebral body. *Spine.* 1981; 6: 217-232.

33. Adams M. Mechanical function of the lumbar apothecial joints. *Spine.* 1983; 8: 327-330.

34. Bogduk N, Twomey L. *Clinical Anatomy of the Lumbar Spine.* Melbourne: Churchill Livingstone; 1987: 60.

35. Tyrell AR, Reilly T, Troup JD. Circadian variations in stature and the effects of spinal loading. *Spine.* 1985; 10: 161-164.

36. Cyriax J. *Textbook of Orthopedic Medicine.* 10th ed. London:

Bailliere Tinda U; 1980: 304.

37. Ramos G. Effects of vertebral axial decompression on intradiscal pressure. *Journal of Neurological Science.* 1994; 81: 350-353.

38. Twomey L. Sustained lumbar traction: An experimental study of long spine segments. *Spine.* 1985; 10: 146-149.

39. Adams M, Bogduk N, Burton K, Dolan P. *Biomechanics of Back Pain.* Edinburgh: Churchill Livingstone; 2002: 27.

40. Lumsden RMD, Morris JM. In vivo study of axial rotation and immobilization at the lumbosacral joint. *Journal of Bone Joint Surgery.* 1968; 50A: 1591.

41. Pearcy M, Tibrewal SB. Axial rotation and lateral bending in the normal lumbar spine measured by three dimensional radiography. *Spine.* 1984; 9: 582-587.

42. White AA, Punjabi *MM. Clinical Biomechanics of the Spine.* 2nd ed. Philadelphia: Lippincott-Raven; 1990.

43. Stokes IA, Wilder DG, Frymoyer JW. Assessment of patients with low back pain by bi-planar radiographic measurement of intervertebral motion. *Spine.* 1981; 6: 233-240.

44. Pearcy M, Portek I, Shepherd J. Three dimensional X-ray analysis of normal movement of the lumbar spine. *Spine.* 1984; 9: 294.

45. Bishop JB, et al. Classification of low back pain from dynamic motion characteristics using an artificial neural network. *Spine.* 1997; 22: 2991-2998.

46. Donelson R, April C, Medcalf R, Grant W. A prospective study of centralization of lumbar and referred pain. *Pain Medical Journal.* 1997; 3: 246-248.

47. Aspen, R. The spine as an arch: a new mathematical model. *Spine.* 1989; 14: 266-274.

48. Armstrong JR. Lumbar disc lesions. *Physiotherapy.* 1964; 50: 284-288.

49. Baretlink DL. Role of abdominal pressure in relieving the pressure on the lumbar intervertebral disks. *Journal of Bone and Joint Surgery.* 1957; 39B: 718-725.

50. Nachemson A. Advances in low back pain. *Clinical Orthopedics.* 1985; 200: 266-278.

51. White AA, Punjabi MM. *Clinical Biomechanics of the Spine.* 2nd ed. Philadelphia: Lippincott-Raven; 1990: 352.

52. Knutsson F. The instability associated with disk degeneration in the lumbar spine. *Acta Radiology.* 1944; 25: 593-609.

53. Punjabi *MM.* The stabilizing system of the spine, part I: function, dysfunction, adaptation, and enhancement. *Journal of Spinal Disorders.* 1992; 5: 383-389.

54. McGill S. *Law Back Disorders.* Champaign, DL: Human Kinetics; 2002: 146.

55. Fritz JM. Segmental instability of the lumbar spine. *Law Back Pain: APTA Monograph.* 1998:152.

V

MECHANICAL DISORDERS
OF THE LUMBOSACRAL SPINE

Back pain can arise within the musculoskeletal system due to muscle strains, ligamentous sprains, inflammation or abnormalities of discs or other spinal structures. It is intermittent and varies with the physical activity. When bending, lifting, twisting or axial loading causes pain, a mechanical disorder is indicated.

Kellagreen demonstrated that noxious stimulation of the low back muscles and interspinous ligaments caused low back pain.[1] And Steindler et al. showed that the cause could be any pathological process that stimulates the nociceptive neurons in the muscles and ligaments involved, and anesthetizing these structures relieves the low back pain.[2]

Sources of noxious stimulation may be either chemical or mechanical. Chemical stimulation occurs due to inflammation and tissue damage. Mechanical stimulation occurs due to irritation when excessive stretching of a ligament puts an array of collagen fibers under tension. This deforms and closes the available space between individual fibers, squeezing them and stimulating the nerve endings within.

For the patient with low back pain, a prompt, thorough clinical evaluation is essential. This includes a carefully detailed, standard history and a complete physical examination according to the Modified Kraus-Weber technique as further modified by one of the authors (CKF) and applied in his practice since 1969 (Chapter 6). This is followed by whatever additional laboratory and radiological tests are needed to clarify or confirm the clinical diagnosis. If the neurological signs are negative and tests for strain/sprain are positive, the patient is diagnosed accordingly and treated as indicated.

With early, accurate diagnosis, the majority of patients with low back pain can be treated with excellent results. Many are thereby prevented from developing low back conditions that would otherwise become chronic. This senior author agrees with those who maintain that accurate diagnosis is possible for the majority of patients with low back pain.

In the 2000 presidential address to the International Society for the study of the Lumbar Spine, Nordin asserts that "We can prevent long-term disability for patients with nonspecific low back pain."[3] But nonspecific back pain, according to the Quebec Task Force Report (QTFR), includes intervertebral disc herniations! This senior author disagrees with the thesis behind the QTFR, specifically the jettisoning of pathology-based diagnoses. Although it was considered a landmark in its time, the QTFR today is considerably out-of-date.[4] The original concern of the Commission was the continual increase in physiotherapy treatments in Quebec, which had risen to 641,197 in 1982."[5]

Wiesel et al. studied 5,362 patients in their clinic with low back pain of unknown etiology.[6] The majority were given definite diagnoses for primary back disorders including back strain, herniated nucleus pulposus and spondylolisthesis. A subgroup of patients were diagnosed as having systemic medical problems including tumors, symptomatic arthritis, ankylosing spondylitis, kidney disease, gall bladder disease and gynecologic pathology. Another subgroup was diagnosed as having psychosocial problems, mainly depression or alcoholism. They found that 98% of the patients, most of whom were given a specific diagnosis, recovered. Of the 2% who either failed to improve with treatment or could not be diagnosed, 10% were found to have a major medical problem.

Wiesel and many others, including Finch and Thompson, do not agree with the all too often stated idea that 85-90% of low back patients cannot be diagnosed.[7, 8] This is incorrect and detrimental to patient care. Even with the existing limitations in tissue-based diagnosis, the diagnostic approach is entirely appropriate and relevant to effective manual/medical treatment and rehabilitation; it must not be neglected in favor of psychosocial approaches.[9]

BACK STRAIN/SPRAIN

Back strains and sprains are a major cause of low back pain and disability among both athletes and industrial workers. In contact sports and athletic activities such as gymnastics, weightlifting, wrestling, golf and rowing, back strains and sprains are common. And among the working population, those who are particularly susceptible to strains and sprains include dock workers, nurses' aides, truck drivers, and others whose jobs require heavy lifting, flexing and twisting motions.

Patients with strains or sprains usually characterize their back pains as spasms or aches. They may be limited to small local areas of the back or may be spread over a large or diffuse area of the lumbar spine with referred pain to the buttocks and posterior thigh.

Seventy percent of patients with back pain experience some

referral of pain to the legs. This referred pain comes from the mesenchymal structures in the lower back, buttocks and posterior thigh that originate from the same embryonic tissue, and is not due to compression of the nerve root, or sciatica. The pain can come from the fascia, muscles, ligaments, periosteum, facet joints, disc or epidural structures and is not referred below the knee. Usually it is a poorly localized, dull pain and may sometimes radiate to both legs.

When this series of events takes place within the muscles, therapists and doctors must take particular care in evaluating the patient; it is easy to jump to the wrong conclusions whenever referred pain is involved.

Prognosis

Strains and sprains are divided into three categories according to prognoses:

1) Mild. Patients have subjective complaints but no objective findings and are able to return to their usual daily activities in less than 10 days.

2) Moderate. Patients complain of pain on palpation, local tenderness with muscle spasms. Range of motion in the spine is limited. With physical therapy, patients can return to their usual daily activities within 14-20 days.

3) Severe. Besides the signs and symptoms of the moderate category, these patients may also exhibit sciatic scoliosis and forward flexion. Their gait is antalgic. Great care must be taken with these patients or their condition may continue to deteriorate, leading to early disc disease. Preparing these patients to resume their usual activities can usually begin after 3-4 weeks of treatment, but any significant low back strain or sprain requires a minimum of 6-8 weeks to heal.

Most back strain and sprain patients improve over a two week period and almost 90% are cured in two months.[10] The 10% who continue to experience low back pain probably were not treated long enough. Using laser endoscopy, tissue pathology not previously visible can now be seen and new studies indicate that less than three months of treatment is insufficient to complete a transformation of fiber type visible at the protein level." The senior author feels that this problem is one of poor diagnosis, poor treatment of acute pain, poor management and poor education both of therapists and patients.

Prompt and appropriate treatment of acute low back strain/sprain, based on proper diagnosis, prevents the development of additional causes of back pain. The first episode of backache is the easiest to treat and the least severe. A second episode lasts longer and is more painful. When the backache is work-related, 60% of the time there is a second episode within a year. Within 3-5 years, the rate may be as high as 50-60%.[12]

MUSCLE STRAINS

Intramuscular pressure increases prodigiously during contraction of the erector spinae muscle, from a resting value of 8 mm of Hg to 265 mm of Hg. Too much tension, too much stretching or a combination of both can indirectly injure the myotendinous unit, leading to muscle strain and pain and damaging fibers.

In their early work on muscle strains, Almikinders and Garrett saw changes in the muscles, but not in the tendons. Possible reasons for this, they speculate, are the slightly increased collagen content of the tendons which decreases their local extensibility, or the increase in sarcomeres near the musculotendinous junction.[14]

There is new evidence that injury to skeletal muscle fibers may occur during isometric contractions, or lengthening contractions (eccentric work).[15, 16] McCully et al. reported a 3-5% loss in the number of fibers when the decrease in force was 50%.[15] To support indirect evidence of muscle damage such as enzyme release from muscle fibers, as well as increased calcium influx, direct measurements of damage to muscle fibers should be proven. An important indirect measure of muscle damage in humans is muscle soreness.[17]

It is now believed that the initial injury to muscle is one of mechanical nature, the sarcomeres being stretched beyond overlap during lengthening contractions. These initial sarcomere injuries are seen in electron micrographs as crumpling of the interface between thick and thin filaments and the disorganization of the Z lines. Following this initial injury, secondary injury takes place depending on the blood supply to the area that is damaged. If the blood supply is impaired then an ischemic reaction follows, while the muscle fibers may remain a necrotic mass of non-contractile tissue which will eventually be infiltrated by fat and connective tissue. On the other hand, if the muscle fibers are adequately supplied by a capillary bed, then a cascade of events involving macrophages and phagocytes infiltrate the area. This leads to secondary injury, causing an inflammatory response. Most fibers may present losses of 50% in maximum force production from 1-3 days after contraction-induced injury. At 14 days they improve to as much as 80% of maximum force production. It is presumed that depending on the severity of the injury, full recovery of normal function takes 7-30 days.[15,17] In humans, according to one theory, rigorous exercise causes micro tears in muscle fibers. The damaged area attracts satellite cells (stem cells) which incorporate themselves into the muscle tissue and begin the process of transcription. The whole process of producing a protein from a gene is called expression of that gene.[16]

Evaluation and Diagnosis

When patients complain of back pain in a local area or in a diffuse area of the lumbar spine, sometimes with the pain radiating to the buttocks or posterior thigh, muscle strain is diagnosed. A traumatic event may cause localized back pain, and tenderness midline or outside the midline on palpation, with muscle spasms and without neurological symptoms. The tenderness is usually off the midline either unilaterally or bilaterally. Sometimes the pain increases in intensity a few hours after the injury. Flexion or extension of the spine is painful due to edema of the structures involved and reflex inhibition of the muscles causes both pain and stiffness.

Since the injured muscles are painful on contraction, the test to confirm this type of injury is to actively contract the muscle against resistance. If this causes pain, the muscle is strained. For example, the suspected presence of a strained erector spinae is confirmed if extension of the lumbar spine against resistance causes pain. Flexing the lumbar spine stretches the erector spinae muscles and after the first 40 degrees of flexion, the stretching also causes pain. So a second test to confirm the injury is to stretch the strained muscle.

Muscle strains are classified according to the severity of the injury into three stages:

Stage 1— microscopic disruption of muscle fiber

Stage 2 — microscopic disruption of muscle fiber but with intact structural integrity of the muscle

Stage 3- complete disruption of the muscle

Muscles examined immediately after injury reveal localized hemorrhage at the muscle/tendon junction. This is also seen 24 hours after injury when the muscles can generate only 50% of their pre-injury force and again at 48 hours, when damage to fibers can be seen.

Histologic examination during the first 24 hours reveals rupture of the muscle fibers close to the myotendinous junction and the presence of inflammation with limited muscle necrosis, leucocyte activity, edema and hemorrhage.

Prognosis

Injury of paraspinal muscles deconditions them, decreasing their mass and the mass of the psoas muscles as well, as seen in radiographs.[18] Decreased muscle mass leads to decreased muscle power (due to atrophy) and this atrophy puts patients at risk of further injury.

During the first 24 and 48 hours after injury, pain and inflammation cause a loss of function. At the end of 7 days, no hemorrhage is seen, and muscles can generate over 90% of their pre-injury force.

In animal studies, gross examination shows a marked reduction in inflammatory activity and fibrosis at the injury site 7 days after injury.[19]

Human patients also regain function after 30 days but during the healing process, fibrosis and development of inelastic scar tissue make recurrence of injuries possible.[19]

Treatment

Muscle strain injuries are managed conservatively, as are Grade 1 and Grade 2 ligamentous sprains. Proper care is crucial from the early acute stage on. As a rule, activity causes pain and rest provides relief.

1. To reduce pain during the acute stage, defined as 30 days or less, and to reduce spasms in muscle strains, most authorities consider the treatment of choice to be cryotherapy followed by Ultrasound (US) to the affected muscle or ligament. Deep friction also can be helpful during the acute stage. During the subacute (30-90 days) stage of strains and sprains, superficial heating with hot packs is beneficial. These treatment techniques are described in Chapter 7. This study showed that patients with non-specific low back pain returned to normal activities, and was superior to the medications mentioned.

2. To increase range of motion, strength, endurance and flexibility, patients are given various exercises. Isometric exercises are given first. Usually patients are comfortable enough to begin 2-3 days after cryotherapy, US and deep friction treatments. Isotonic exercises are given next, then strength, endurance and flexibility exercises, always within the patient's pain tolerance. The exercises are described in Chapter 7.

3. To prepare the patient gradually to resume normal daily activities, work and sports, usually after about 3-4 weeks (subacute stage), counseling is necessary. Most patients need to make appropriate changes in the manner in which they perform their ordinary everyday actions involved in living, working and playing to avoid misuse of the back. See Chapter 7.

At this time, athletes and those with occupational injuries are well advised to take up additional strength, endurance and flexibility exercises such as swimming, stationary bicycling and leg pressing to maintain cardiovascular health and muscle tone.

LIGAMENTOUS SPRAINS

Disruptions of ligmentous connections between bones are termed sprains and they also can cause low back pain.

Evaluation

Since ligaments are inert and do not contract as do muscles, sprains must be tested passively. Stiffness and tenderness are found on palpation; midline tenderness is often found in interspinous ligaments. Except for the supraspinous ligaments, these structures lie deep in the back and patients develop back pain that may be difficult to diagnose. With supraspinous ligament sprain, patients feel midline tenderness on palpation and pain on passive flexion of the lumbar spine. A suspected sprain in a certain ligament is confirmed if passively stressing that ligament causes pain.

Sprains are categorized according to severity into four grades:

(Grade 1) partial tears with no defect or instability,

(Grade 2) a palpable defect but no instability,

(Grade 3) subluxation of the facet joint with no dislocation,

(Grade 4) complete ligamentous disruption and dislocation.

Treatment

Ligamentous sprains in grades 1 and 2 are managed conservatively, the same as muscle strain injuries. Ligamentous sprains in grades 3 and 4 are treated surgically.

Muscle Spasms

Various problems can cause muscle spasms and patients cannot all be treated the same way. In some patients with low back pain, constant contraction of the paraspinal muscles can produce muscle spasms. Borenstein and Weisel reason that these spasms may be due to an absence of blood flow resulting in an accumulation of metabolic byproducts, which could stimulate pain receptors within blood vessels.[20]

Findings are mixed regarding EMG activity in patients with muscle spasms in their backs. Some authors, Cooper for one, demonstrated increased EMG activity in such muscles.[21] Others have found no EMG activity in muscle spasms.[22] During the course of many EMG studies of patients referred clinically, this senior author has seen SEMG activity in muscle spasms and found that a critical determinant is the patient's position while being tested.[23] If the patient is lying down, SEMG values are normal; if the patient is sitting, the side with the spasms shows SEMG activity.

During the acute stage of low back pain, muscle spasms may belong to one of two types. In Type 1 spasms, the pain-spasm-pain cycle postulated by Travell and supported by Roland[24, 25], myoelectric activity using SEMG, is silent in these patients, but on palpation, the muscle is hard to the touch. Ultrasound must not be used on these patients since it could increase the blood flow to the area, causing a venous occlusion in the intervertebral foramen, resulting in ischemia and more pain. For these patients, the senior author uses interferential therapy (IT) to minimize pain and produce a pumping action helpful in venous stasis. Causes of this type of spasm are muscle strain, accumulation of anaerobic metabolic byproducts and a compartment syndrome, which is very rare. Treatment of choice is ice packs every few hours followed by IT, and when pain subsides, exercises. With this treatment, the problem usually disappears. The senior author recently treated a young woman about 34 years of age, a professional golfer with this syndrome. She had played a round of golf and then did pushups in her hot tub. The next morning she was in severe pain, unable to move. The same day he treated her with cold packs and IT. In three days, she felt normal.

Type 2 is muscle spasm in acute low back pain patients; myoelectric activity is high with SEMG (over 5 microvolts) and the muscles are hard on palpation. Patients have a scoliotic list as a protective mechanism. This type of muscle spasm is often due to an early disc lesion, which clearly demonstrates why all patients with low back pain cannot be lumped together and treated alike.

Muscle Fatigue

Muscle fatigue, associated with overuse, abuse and misuse can cause muscle pain. Muscle fatigue increases concentration of lactic acid which causes pain and releases inflammatory mediators associated with muscle edema, another cause of pain. This theory seems to be no longer tenable. Pedersen et al.[26] challenge this traditional view. They demonstrated that lactic acid, in fact, has beneficial effects on performance of fatigued muscles. They show in rat muscle fiber preparations that lactic acid influences the activity of chloride ion channels, which helps to sustain the action potentials that are necessary for muscle contraction. Nielsen and his colleagues helped us understand the effects of muscle acidosis.[27] They showed that accumulation of extra-cellular potassium ions was the main reason for muscle fatigue, and showed that force in an isolated muscle declined sharply when the potassium concentration increased. They also showed that if the muscle was rendered acidic, much of the lowered force was reversed and was accompanied by recovery of action potential generation.[27]

Overuse of back muscles and muscle fatigue impair precise motor control, as is well documented, and has a deleterious effect in the work place.[26, 29, 30] Myoelectric evidence has demonstrated muscle fatigue among workers subjected to whole-body vibration, such as truck drivers, heavy laborers, dock workers and cement workers. Athletes too, if poorly trained in how to avoid muscle fatigue, may suffer debilitating effects in their performance. In a fatigued condition, the resulting loss of contractility leads to muscle strain and loss of energy absorption.

Low back problems that involve the multifidus muscle and other conditions such as tennis elbow make muscles and tendons more prone to fatigue failure.

Injuries in the Multifidus Triangle

The multifidus triangle, which is bound by the area lateral to the fourth and fifth lumbar vertebra, and medial to the posterior iliac crest, contains many muscles, like the multifidus and the quadratus lumborum, and many ligaments, like the transverse ligament, iliolumbar ligament and the dorsolumbar fascia. This area is susceptible to low back injuries, as reported by Bauwens, due to the fact that much stress is placed in this area of the lumbosacral spine.[31]

Ruptured Tendons

Tendons, the fibrous bands that connect muscles to bones, are mainly composed of wavy, parallel collagen fibers with elastin fibers in between and the bulk provided by reticulin fibers. These fiber components are suspended in a gelatinous substance that reduces friction between them. Tendons have twice the tensile strength of muscles and contraction of the muscle does not rupture the tendon even if as much as 50% of it is severed.[32] When a tendon is exposed to a physiologic load that exceeds its yield point, its components rupture. Collagen does not rupture until stretched to 6-8 times its length, but elastin is brittle compared to collagen, and ruptures when stretched to twice its original length. When a tendon ruptures, capillaries are disrupted, causing a clot to form and healing takes place with scar tissue. Scarring stiffens the musculotendinous unit, causing it to operate at a disadvantage. The repair process of tendons is similar to that of muscles.

Scarring

When muscles and tendons heal with scar tissue, they lose compliance and their efficiency is diminished. Prevention of injuries, therefore, is a better strategy than treatment. However, once an injury occurs, competent therapy can help compensate for muscular hypertrophy and thickening of tendons.

One goal of physical therapy is to limit the formation of scar tissue and to preserve the contractility and strength of muscles and the elasticity of tendons.

Myofascial Pain Syndrome

Often associated with minor strains or sprains, myofascial pain syndrome is not accompanied by motor or neurological symptoms.[33] To many authorities, it is low back pain with no structural defect and accounts for nearly 85-90% of cases of low back pain.[34] Some authors claim that as many as 94% of cases of low back pain are called "nonspecific" or "strain-sprain" because the cause is unknown.[35]

The presence of trigger points differentiates myofascial low back pain from other low back pain. Mechanical, repetitive strain at these points is believed to cause myofascial pain.[36, 37]

Soft Tissue Injuries

Fewer than 10% of all musculoskeletal injuries are soft tissue injuries. Sprains and strains such as occur among athletes account for most soft tissue injuries. Persons in occupations that involve heavy labor, like dock workers and cement workers, and those involved in motor vehicle accidents, also suffer these injuries.

Prompt and competent treatment is crucial for acute patients, since these injuries can lead to further mechanical problems such as disc disease and spinal stenosis. Correct therapy early on reduces the need for back surgery.

Lumbar Compartment Syndrome

The lumbar compartment is interiorly bound by the transverse processes and the intertransverse ligaments; it is dorsally and laterally bounded by the lumbodorsal fascia and medially by the vertebra and discs. Carr et al. studied the pressures within this closed compartment with subjects in various positions and recorded pressures during normal breathing and during valsalva maneuvers.[38] Some authorities doubt this proposition.[39]

Physiologically, two types of lumbar pain syndrome can be identified: (1) the Somatic Pain syndrome in which the pain is directly attributed to the musculoskeletal structures of the lumbar spine, and (2) the Radicular Pain syndrome in which the pain is due to disorders of the spinal nerves or the spinal nerve roots.

INTERVERTEBRAL DISC CONDITIONS

In describing intervertebral discs, it is essential that therapists involved in clinical, diagnostic and therapeutic procedures use standard terminology to describe both normal and pathologic conditions. This is particularly crucial when communicating impressions gleaned from imaging in order to be understood and interpreted with reasonably consistent accuracy and precision. For this reason, the Combined Task Forces of the North American Spine Society, the American Society of Spine Radiology and the American Society of Neuroradiology have recommended the classification of disc conditions as developed by Fardon.[40]

Normal discs are young and have no morphological abnormalities. The development of a central band of fibrous tissue resulting in a bilocular appearance is considered normal. **Congenital/Developmental variations** are discs that have undergone changes due to abnormal growth of the spine as in scoliosis or spondylolisthesis.

Degenerative/Traumatic changes include annular tears, herniations and degeneration. Neither trauma, nor pathologic degenerative conditions, are necessary conditions.

Bulging Discs occur when disc tissue extends beyond the edges of the apophyses — usually less than *3mm* beyond the edges. In a bulging disc, the periphery of the annulus extends beyond the margin delineated by the vertebral body end plates. But unlike a herniated disc, which is always associated with a disrupted annulus, a budging disc still contains its focal material within the outer walls of the annulus.

Protruding Disc or Contained Herniation occurs when discal material — nuclear, annular or end plate — is displaced beyond the normal peripheral margins of the disc. The normal peripheral margin of the disc is limited by adjacent vertebral body end plates. In addition, the outer annulus is not breached and the discal material remains beneath the outer layer of the annulus. It is distinguished from a bulging disc based on the shape of the displaced discal material. A disc is protruded if the greater plane between the edges of the disc tissue beyond the disc space in any direction is less than the distance between the edges of the base measured in the same plane.

Extruded Disc occurs when discal material has broken through the outer annulus. It may or may not remain beneath the posterior longitudinal ligament (PLL); it is called an extrusion. If the disc is contained by the PLL it is called a sub-ligamentous extrusion. If the disc has penetrated the PLL and lies in the epidural space, it is called a transligamentous extrusion. If extruded material breaks away, is not in contact with the original discal substance and is lying beneath the PLL, then it is called sequestrated or free.

Herniated Disc occurs when localized discal material — nucleus pulposus, cartilage, fragmented apophyseal bone, or fragmented annular tissue — is displaced beyond the space of the intervertebral disc. Displacement via the end plates as in Schmorl's nodes is called intravertebral herniation.

As far back as 1974 it was apparent to this senior author that most patients referred to therapy with a diagnosis of low back pain of unknown etiology, with diffuse back pain but no pain radiating to the lower extremities, could well be suffering from herniated discs. They were undiagnosed since they could only be detected by discography.[41] Even without the availability of MRIs and CT Scans, with the help of history taking and clinical evaluation, these patients could be diagnosed, effectively treated and the need for surgery minimized. Today, many experts agree that in the vast majority of cases, back pain and radiating pain indicate a disc problem. And although it has not been proven, the evidence of recent anatomic studies and discography suggests that as many as 80% of all low back syndromes relate to the lumbar disc.[42]

During the course of a herniated disc, 80% of patients experience significant back pain, but only 35% develop true sciatica, which may develop 6-10 years after the onset of low back pain. During this period repeated damage to annular fibers may irritate the sinuvertebral nerve without causing sciatica.[43]

Horwitz, as early as 1939, in a report on 75 cadavers, found 50 posterior bulges without herniations among 50 of the specimens studied. In radiography studies of 409 lumbar discs, Horwitz found 119 normal discs, 184 posterior hernias and 117 other hernias (lateral, anterior and vertical).[44]

Clearly, scientists or anatomists were making correct diagnoses before CT Scans and MRIs were available.

Natural History of Disc Degeneration

Our understanding of disc degeneration is based on a combination of retrospective and prospective studies using various criteria such as clinical signs, symptoms and radiological evidence.

In one study, disc degeneration began among persons in their teens, and by twenty years of age, the frequency of degeneration and protrusion increased and remained unchanged, respectively. They found that low back pain was most likely to persist among those individuals who showed the first signs of disc degeneration.[45]

A study by Weber also showed that the first attacks of low back pain occurred among persons in their twenties, and ten years later, the first radicular signs appeared.[46] This author attributes the first attack of lumbago and the onset of radiating pain to intradiscal degeneration, with the greatest risk of disabling sciatica at about forty years of age.

Saal et al. observed 64 patients with verified disc herniation and radiculopathy who were treated conservatively.[47] After a year, 90% had improved satisfactorily. Treatments consisted of physiotherapeutic interventions, NSAIDs and epidural steroid injections. The physical treatments included ice packs, body mechanics to facilitate pain-free movement, back extension exercises, traction, TENS and acupuncture.

Pathophysiology

Younger individuals with a mean age of thirty-five years have the highest risk of developing herniations of intervertebral discs.[48,49]

Most disc problems occur at L5-S1 and L4-L5. These are the two most common levels of herniation and together they account for 95% of all lumbar disc herniations.

Posterolateral herniations, the most common position of herniations, affect the nerve root at the level beneath the herniation; L4-L5 herniation affects the L5 root and L5-S1 herniation affects the S1 root. Foraminal and extraforaminal herniations may affect the nerve root exiting at the same level, e.g. L4-L5 herniation may affect the L4 root.

Upper lumbar disc herniations are not common. They seldom occur at L4-L3 and L3-L2. Herniations at L3-L4 account for fewer than 2-3% of all lumbar disc herniations and affect the L4 nerve root. Fewer than 5% of all disc herniations occur above L4; of these, 83% are at L3-L4.[50] In diagnosing upper lumbar disc herniations, the femoral nerve stretching test is a valuable sign. It is important to remember that back pain and pain radiating anteriorly down the upper thigh may be due to either L3-L4 disc herniations or to foraminal and extraforaminal disc herniations of the L3-L4 disc. The femoral and crossed femoral stretch are positive in either case. This maneuver, by stretching the femoral nerve in the psoas and quadriceps muscles, applies direct traction to the upper lumbar nerve roots, according to Dyck.[51]

The symptoms when a lower lumbar disc is herniated are caused by both biochemical and mechanical inflammation of nerve roots.

Although not yet proved, fragmentation of the disc probably precedes annular rupture, as most authorities believe. Disc fragmentation has been shown in adolescents to begin with dehydration, intradiscal fissuring and degeneration followed by disruption of the inner annulus, then the outer, thereby causing annular tear with resulting disc herniation. Because only the inner annulus, which is not innervated, is involved, there is no pain. During the period affecting the outer annulus, the outer third of which is innervated and pain sensitive, the patient complains of back pain. Finally, with herniation of the disc, the nerve root is affected and the patient complains of sharp, lacerating pain. This is the characteristic radicular pain that defines sciatica.

Interestingly, once a disc ruptures, the patient no longer has back pain. Radicular pain replaces the back pain, because when the disc ruptures, its contents are extruded into the spinal canal, reducing the painful pressure inside the disc. In many instances, a patient can be asymptomatic throughout the entire process. The size of the canal — whether there is enough space for both the disc and the nerve root — is the determining factor.[52] A minor herniation in a small canal may be crippling because there isn't enough room for both disc and nerve root, while a major herniation in a large canal may be asymptomatic.

Any flexion movements of the spine cause pain, while extension movements relieve it. As a rule, coughing, sneezing or straining during bowel movements all exacerbate the pain of herniated discs.

To conceptualize disc degeneration, protrusion and herniation, various studies have been performed. A convincing study by Moore et al.[53] showed that herniation is a result of migration of nuclear fragments through previously existing defects in the annulus. They found that the migratory fragments were predominantly nuclear, with a small amount of annular material, mainly from the inner, transitional zone.[53]

According to some authorities, repeated activities putting low loads on the spine cause chronic mechanical fatigue of annular fibers, progressing to prolapse.[54] Other authorities believe that shearing forces create radiating clefts in the annular fibers.[55] Most agree that degenerative changes appear in the nucleus by the second decade of life. And after a traumatic event, even in the young, the annulus is ruptured and the turgid nucleus is extruded under pressure. Clinically symptomatic disc protrusions are prevalent during middle age and later; it is apparent that the disc nucleus has lost its turgidity and age-related degeneration has caused herniation.

In the studies of Adams and Hutton[56], severely degenerated discs were found not to prolapse.

In these studies, the compressive force required to cause herniation was, on average, 5.4 kN, range *2.8-13.0* kN. The angle of hyperflexion of the motion segment ranged from 9 to 21 degrees. Later studies by the same authors indicated that the flexion angle need not be high provided the compressive forces or the flexion angle exceeded normal, everyday limits.

Another study illustrates the mechanics of a severely degenerated disc prolapse. Posterior disc prolapse was produced in non-degenerated motion segments taken from cadavers 20-52 years of age using up to 6 degrees of flexion and compressive forces of 1-6 kN. The disc was weakened before testing by slicing into an area of the posterior annulus, 10 mm by 10 mm. The outermost 1 mm of annulus, however, was left intact. The nucleus of the disc was replaced with chopped pieces of annulus from another disc to make the disc less turgid.

Lu and Hutton clearly demonstrated that a fully hydrated disc can prolapse and herniate when loads are rapidly applied to the spine, accompanied by axial rotation with bending and compression.[58]

Muscle Spasms, Sciatic List and Herniated Discs

Muscle spasm by itself, whether unilateral or bilateral, is not diagnostic of a disc lesion, but when accompanied by such other signs as sciatic list or sciatic scoliosis, it is fairly indicative of disc herniation.

In a study of 40 consecutive patients with herniations, 29 had a lesion at L4-L5 with L5 radiculopathy and 11 had a herniation at L5-S1 with a S1 radiculopathy.[59]

Persons with low back pain are not significantly different from a normal population in postural anterior-posterior lumbosacral list (lateral deviation), according to Arangio.[60] However, Porter found that 5.6% of patients deviate to some degree away from the painful side.[61] McKenzie, disagreeing with other authorities, states that 56% of patients with low back pain present a sciatic scoliosis, a claim that is, unfortunately, accepted on faith by therapists who subscribe to his techniques of treatment.[62]

It is known that sciatic scoliotic list is related to lumbar disc herniation, but the mechanism and significance of the relationship is not fully understood. The sciatic scoliotic list that accompanies a herniated disc is gravity-dependent; patients with a herniated disc can abolish their list by lying down. Their radiographs at this time will show no scoliosis. Another way they can abolish the list is by hanging from a bar [63]; this is clinically important in conservative treatment. Patients with structural lumbar scoliosis or deformity, on the other hand, cannot affect it by lying down.

Porter et al.[64] believe that sciatic scoliosis is present in 5.6% of patients with a herniated disc, low back pain and spasms. The gravity-dependent list was seen in 100 out of 1776 back patients

(5.6%) at their clinic.[6'''] Some characteristics of this group are interesting to note:

Age	Average 38 years
Sex	62% male, 38% female
List to the left	66 pts
List to the right	31 pts
To both sides	3 pts
Pain	
Back, below the knee, root involvement	71 pts
Back only	16 pts
Back, thigh, not below knee	13 pts

Those with a list and back pain only may have a protruding disc that affects nerve-sensitive areas but not the root.[66] Most of the patients with radicular pain also had a positive test for straight-leg raising (SLR) and showed muscle wasting, weakness and diminished reflexes.[67] Although Porter believes that his conservative treatment would have proven to be better, 40% of the patients in this group were treated surgically.[68]

The McKenzie technique, based on the invalid hypothesis of Finneson regarding sciatic list, is incorrect and for most patients is bound to fail. Finneson held that when the herniation is lateral to the nerve root, the list is toward the opposite side of the sciatica to diminish nerve compression; and when the herniation is at the axilla of the nerve root, the list is toward the same side as the sciatica to decrease the nerve-root compression. Finneson's hypothesis is no longer tenable based on recent studies, mainly those of Matsui et al.[69]

Studies of Matsui et al. show that at any topographic location of disc herniation, the sciatic scoliotic list is apt to occur with the convexity to the symptomatic side of the herniation.[70] The list disappeared completely in 18 of the 40 patients these authors studied, most frequently among those with herniations medial to the nerve root or in the axilla. The list persisted longer among those with herniations lateral to the nerve root.[71]

The sciatic scoliotic list, which is also a protective spasm, may be elucidated in the work of Hirayama, Tiro et al.[72] In patients with lumbar radiculopathy, it may be induced by a spinal reflex due to pain from an injured spinal root. Pain could produce changes in the asymmetric excitability of spinal neurons relating to the postural reflex, leading to asymmetric trunk muscle tonus.[73]

Structural scoliotic list can be differentiated from a nonstructural sciatic scoliotic list in two ways. (1) The structure of the vertebral column and thoracic ribs are asymmetric in forward flexion and the shoulder is elevated on the convex side of the scoliotic curve. When the scoliosis is nonstructural, no asymmetry and no structural anatomic changes in the vertebra and ribs are seen on forward flexion. Also, a nonstructural scoliosis is in the lumbar region and has its apex in the same region. (2) In a structural scoliotic list, the lumbar lordosis is obliterated; these patients have a flat back.

The senior author does SEMG studies with these patients. When prone, those with a sciatic scoliosis due to a disc lesion will disappear, and SEMG on both sides are within normal limits (less than 5 microvolts). In patients with structural scoliosis, however, the scoliosis will not disappear when prone, and on the scoliotic side the SEMG will be over 5 microvolts. When sitting, the patients with a sciatic scoliosis will have increased electrical activity on SEMG tests, with the side of the convexity well over 5 microvolts.[74]

The clinical protocol includes history-taking, observation, examination and special tests of reflexes, joint movements and muscle strength. Specific test procedures are detailed in Chapter

6 and specific treatments in Chapter 7.

Patient history includes a complete medical history emphasizing areas of clinical relevance. Important data are age, occupation, onset of the problem, whether gradual or sudden, whether similar episodes occurred in the past, at what intervals and whether traumatic. Regarding the pain, note whether it is constant, intermittent or occasional. Is it at one location or does it radiate? Is it associated with rest, certain postures, certain movements, at certain times of day?

The characteristic quality of the pain must be determined. Nerve pain is sharp, bright and burning; it usually radiates along the nerve. Bone pain is deep, boring and very localized. Muscle pain is diffused aching, often hard to localize and may be referred to other parts of the body. Muscle pain may be aggravated by injury.

A herniated disc can be identified by some of the patients' answers to questions about their pain. The pain due to a herniated disc is sharp, burning, stabbing. Its onset may be gradual but more often is sudden and radiates down the leg on a dermatome, usually extending below the knee with sensations of pins and needles and tingling. Some patients describe pain along with tingling and numbness in the anterior part of the thigh. Certain movements such as standing up from a sitting position or sitting for long periods can cause pain. Bowel movements can cause pain. All patients complain of severe pain on coughing and sneezing. Such pains are associated with increased intradiscal pressure. Spinal flexion activities increase the pain for most patients while spinal extension relieves it. Rest relieves the pain for most patients.

When sciatica develops fully and radiates fully down the buttocks, thigh and leg in its dermatomal distribution, the back pain sometimes disappears, since the annulus has ruptured, minimizing intradiscal pressure.

Distinguishing radicular pain from referred pain is important and determines how to treat the patient. Many therapists incorrectly believe that pain below the knee is radicular and pain above the knee is referred. This simplistic dichotomy can lead therapists to wrong treatment decisions and unhappy patients to unnecessary surgeries.

Radicular pain occurs when axons of a spinal nerve or neurons in the dorsal root ganglion are irritated. Referred pain, on the other hand, occurs when nociceptive free nerve endings in somatic or visceral tissue are activated. A common example is pain in the arm caused by an ischemic heart condition. Physiologically, afferent neurons converge onto common neurons in the central nervous system (CNS), which may be unable to distinguish the source of this input of referred pain.[75]

Pain is often assumed to be radicular when imaging studies show disc herniation and nerve-root compression, as many studies confirm.[75] It has been suggested that some patients' leg pain may be referred pain from small, contained herniations or bulges where the degree of nerve-root compression is small compared to that of extrusions and sequestrations.

Conor et al. experimentally demonstrated beyond a doubt that noxious stimulation of the disc can produce referred pain below the knee similar to radicular pain.[76] Naturally occurring noxious stimulation due to chemical or mechanical events in the disc can do the same. This is seen in cases of noxious stimulation secondary to pathologic disc lesions without nerve-root compression.

Treatment strategies, whether conservative, as in physical therapy, or surgical, differ for referred and radicular pain as mentioned, hence the importance of differentiating them. Such clinical tests as the straight-leg-raising (SLR) test make differential diagnosis possible; dorsiflexion of the foot above 40 degrees causes no pain in cases of referred pain.

Physical Evaluation

This author has used a modified Kraus-Weber test (Chapter 6) for all low back pain patients since 1969. This includes sensitive and specific clinical tests for low back pain that are, even today, more specific and sensitive than those proposed by the NIOSH task force.[77] A test is said to be sensitive when it correctly detects the problem in patients. It is said to be specific when it correctly reveals the absence of the problem in the patients. Ideally, diagnostic tests should be positive for all patients who have the disease and negative for all who are free of it.[78]

This senior author uses nine tests with the patient standing and lying down (Chapter 6). Performed carefully and properly, these tests and any indicated EMGs and MRIs confirm the diagnosis, paving the way for appropriate treatments. This approach has proven competent, safe and effective over the years, unlike the highly questionable guidelines issued by the Agency for Health Care Policy and Research (AHCPR) which conclude with the absurd advice that for acute low back pain, the only acceptable treatments are rest and exercise.[79]

Observation

Not all examiners ask patients to undress to the waist! Some patients have said that their physicians and orthopedic surgeons omitted this important first step! It is necessary to have all low back pain patients undress to the waist in order to see such structural deformities as scoliosis, kyphosis, exaggerated lordosis and obliterated lordosis, or flat back. Otherwise these defects could be missed. Having the patient undress to the waist also makes it possible to see such events as muscle spasms and scoliotic lists with elevated hips on one side. And range of motion (ROM) can be measured in flexion, extension and lateral flexion. These movements may be restricted, and while not diagnostic of disc herniations by themselves, they may later be a measure of patients' progress and improvement.

The Neurologic Examination is most important in acute sciatica, to pinpoint any nerve-root compression. Disc herniations are most common at L4-L5 and L5-S1; together they account for 95% of all herniations and those at L2-L3 and L3-L4 account for fewer than 5%. Ordinarily, sciatica develops 6-10 years after onset of the first episode of back pain, so the early history is important. If the first episode of back pain is correctly treated, patients will not be subjected to second and third episodes and progression to disc herniations, 35% of which culminate in sciatica.

Most tests of nerve roots put them under tension and cause pain or paresthesia. Being mobile, the nerve roots are capable of a certain amount of excursion. The S1 nerve root can move about 4mm, the L5 about the same and the L4 about 3mm. With a herniated disc, the nerve root cannot move freely, hence the pain and paresthesia.

When the S1 nerve root is compressed, the patient complains of weakness and atrophy of the gastrocnemius and is unable to stand on the toes of the foot on the affected side. The Achilles reflex also is diminished or absent. See Figure 10.

When the L5 nerve root is compressed, the extensor halluces longus (EHL) muscle, the long extensor of the great toe, is weakened. Any weakness of this muscle is a sign of L5 root compression. Sensory loss occurs on the anterior surface of the left and the dorsomedial aspect of the foot to the great toe. See Figure 11.

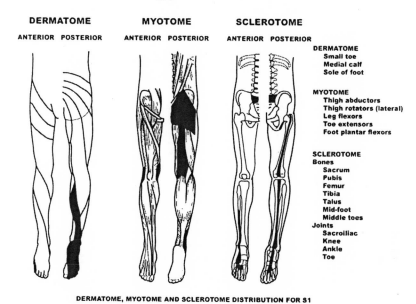

S1

DERMATOME, MYOTOME AND SCLEROTOME DISTRIBUTION FOR S1

Figure 10

When the L4 root is compressed, the knee extensors, or quadriceps are weakened. Patients complain of the knee buckling and atrophy of the muscle. The patella tendon reflex is diminished and sensory loss occurs in the dermatomal pattern. See Figure 12.

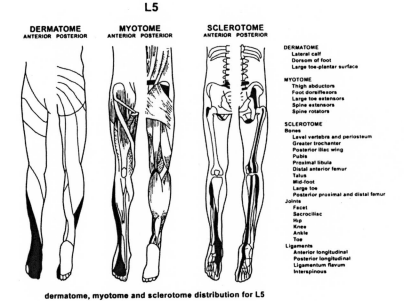

L5

DERMATOME
ANTERIOR POSTERIOR

MYOTOME
ANTERIOR POSTERIOR

SCLEROTOME
ANTERIOR POSTERIOR

DERMATOME
  Lateral calf
  Dorsom of foot
  Large toe-plantar surface

MYOTOME
  Thigh abductors
  Foot dorsiflexors
  Large toe extensors
  Spine extensors
  Spine rotators

SCLEROTOME
Bones
  Level vertebra and periosteum
  Greater trochanter
  Posterior iliac wing
  Pubis
  Proximal fibula
  Distal anterior femur
  Talus
  Mid-foot
  Large toe
  Posterior proximal and distal femur
Joints
  Facet
  Sacroiliac
  Hip
  Knee
  Ankle
  Toe
Ligaments
  Anterior longitudinal
  Posterior longitudinal
  Ligamentum flavum
  Interspinous

dermatome, myotome and sclerotome distribution for L5

Figure 11

L4

DERMATOME
ANTERIOR POSTERIOR

MYOTOME
ANTERIOR POSTERIOR

SCLEROTOME
ANTERIOR POSTERIOR

DERMATOME
  Anterior lower leg
  Lateral knee
  Medial ankle

MYOTOME
  Thigh abductors
  Thigh flexors
  Thigh rotators
  Leg extensors
  Foot dorsiflexors
  Foot supinators
  Spine extensors
  Spine rotators

SCLEROTOME
Bones
  Level vertebra and
    periosteum iliac wing
  Femur (medial and lateral)
  Tibia (medial plateau and
    lateral epicondyle)
  Talus
Joints
  Facet
  Hip
  Knee
  Ankle
Ligaments
  Anterior longitudinal
  Posterior longitudinal
  Ligamentum flavum
  Interspinous

Dermatome, myotome and sclerotome distribution for L4

Figure 12

108

The Lasegue Test, a passive straight-leg-raising (SLR) test, causes pain up to about 70 degrees; pain or tightness beyond that point is due to tight hamstring muscles.[80] The test is performed with the patient prone and lifting the leg, which causes tension in the S1 nerve root. The test is positive when pain is felt below the knee on raising the leg about 70 degrees or if radicular pain continues as before.

The cross-SLR test, or SLR opposite of the symptomatic leg, when positive, that is, giving rise to pain in the affected leg, is suggestive of a massive disc herniation.

Shiqing et al. described the location of the pain in relation to the position of the herniated disc.[81] Central protrusions, they found, caused back pain; lateral protrusions caused pain down the leg; intermediate protrusions caused pain in the leg as well as the back.

Manual tests of muscles

Wasting and weakness of certain muscles are signs of root compression at particular sites. As mentioned, weakness of the extensor halluces longus (EHL) muscle indicates the most common site of herniation, L4-L5. Wasting and weakness of other muscles, and the sites of root compression that they indicate, are as follows:

Weak Muscle	Site of compressed root
EHL	L4-L5
Quadriceps	L2-L4
Anterior tibialis	L4
Extensor Digitorum brevis and longus	L5
Peroneus longus and brevis	S1
Gastrocnemius-soleus	S1-S2
Gluteus maximus	S1
*Gluteus minimus	L5

*tested with patients lying on their sides

Knee and ankle reflexes are routinely tested to determine L4-S1 integrity.

A drop foot could be due either to injury of the peroneal nerve or to an L5 radiculopathy. Differential diagnosis is important since treatments are so different. Weakness of the gluteus maximus and tensor fascia latae indicate an L5 radiculopathy. The Trendelenburg sign is another indication of an L5 radiculopathy. See Table 1

Palpation and Percussion

When the back extensor muscles are bilaterally in spasm, their hardness can be felt when palpated 1-3 cm from the midline.

When spasms are one-sided, a scoliotic list can be seen with the convexity to the contracted side; this is suggestive of a far lateral disc herniation. When standing, the SEMG test will show muscle activity on the convex side while the other side is normal. If the patient is tested when prone, with a pillow under the abdomen, no activity appears on SEMG testing on either side; the sciatic scoliosis will have disappeared. This test is another way to differentiate a structural scoliosis, which does not disappear, from a sciatic list.

Percussion over the lumbar spine may cause local pain or sometimes sciatica in the presence of nerve-root compression; this is only suggestive of disc herniation.

Painful or tender motor points on lower muscles of the affected leg demonstrate their innervation due to nerve root involvement and are probably diagnostic and prognostic of disc herniation, according to Gunn et al.[82] These authors maintain that among patients without radicular pain, those with tender motor points will remain disabled three times as long as those without this sign; and if radiculopathy is present, patients with this sign will be disabled four times as long. Since the test is performed only in special instances at the senior author's clinic, and not as part of the ordinary routine, we cannot confirm this. See Figure 13.

CLINICAL SYNDROME OF LUMBAR DISC DISEASE

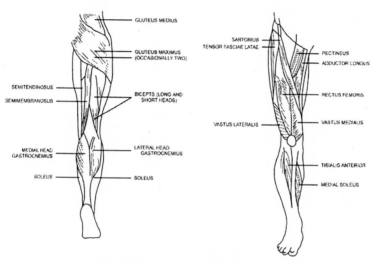

MOTOR POINTS OF THE LOWER EXTREMITIES.
A DIAGNOSTIC AND PROGNOSTIC AID FOR LOW-BACK INJURY

Motor points of the lower extremities. (From Gunn, C.C., Chir, B., and Milbrant, W.E.: Tenderness at motor points: A diagnostic and prognostic aid for low back injury. J. Bone Joint Surg. (Am.) 58:815, 1976.)

Figure 13

Treatment of Intervertebral Disc Diseases

Lumbar disc lesions require treatments unlike those for low back pain due to sprains, making accurate diagnosis essential. Unfortunately, some authors fail to make the distinction. Some studies that exclude patients with pain radiating below the knee generalize their conclusions to include patients with pain due to disc herniations! Two examples are: Deyo et al. and Rozenberg et al.[83, 84] Treating patients with herniated discs the same as those with sprains or strains may account for the explosion in the numbers of surgeries despite the decrease in numbers of cases of low back pain.

Acute pain, as defined by the International Association for the Study of Pain, is pain lasting less than three months (subacute: 30-60 days).[85] Management of acute and subacute low back pain with disc herniations has two objectives: (1) To relieve pain, muscle spasms and inflammation as quickly as possible, and (2) To minimize the possibility of patients becoming chronic, hence alleviating any problems related to chronicity.

Firstly, rest enhances the natural healing of affected structures. In most cases, lumbar herniated discs involve a propulsion of the nucleus pulposus out of the annulus, causing pain due to the chemical effect of substance P, or nitric oxide, and not due to the compression of the nerve root. Since the nucleus pulposus is 90% water, it will be absorbed if allowed to rest. The annulus has a natural, healthy tendency to heal, but if the structures are not allowed rest, the healing is delayed with adverse effects. Deleterious effects of rest, however, must be weighed against its beneficial effects, with the patients fully informed and advised.

Most patients with lumbar disc herniations exhibit muscle spasms, either bilateral or unilateral, depending on the severity of the condition. Palpation alone is insufficient for diagnosis. They may be benign or pathological and the only way to differentiate the two is by surface EMG techniques, which this senior author uses in his practice. Finneson's theory that disc herniations medial to the nerve root deviate away from the midline is no longer tenable.[86] New studies show that 80% of sciatic scoliosis is on the convex side. The use of the lateral wedge maneuver to treat these patients is therefore incorrect both scientifically and theoretically.[87]

Most importantly, patients in severe pain must be cared for with bed rest, pain medications and *any* physical modalities that minimize pain. This senior author uses a combination of interferential therapy, low level laser therapy with ice packs and positioning to make the patient comfortable. The position of choice is the 90/90 position with distraction techniques first advocated by Cortrell.[88] This position effectively reduces intradiscal pressure, as Nachemson[89] demonstrated in his classic studies. The technique is called unloading the lumbar spine. By minimizing muscle activity in the psoas muscle, the position helps lower discal pressure. It also minimizes the stretch on the sciatic nerve. In addition, distraction in this position decompresses any spinal nerve roots that are impinged due to the opening up of the IVF. We now believe that this position also aids nutrition to the disc, hence the position has a salutary effect as well. Our patients are advised to take this position twice a day, remaining in it for thirty minutes each time, as the benefits are enormous.

Always, the patients' pain is the determining factor of treatment type. All the patients' movements must be within the pain-free range. In one of the better studies[90] of low back pain patients, most of them without lumbar disc herniations, one group was allowed four days of complete bed rest initially, while another group was allowed to attend to all their usual daily activities within their pain tolerance and also allowed twelve hours of bed rest daily, including nights. At the end of three months, the two groups were alike.[90] This clinician believes that judicious use of isometric exercises along with bed rest prevents atrophy due to disuse and any other harmful consequences of complete bed rest.

Secondly, to insure against development of a chronic condition, as soon as the patient is comfortable enough, exercises can be started to increase strength, endurance and range of motion.

Building strength

It is well known that the muscles around the lumbar spine are weak and in persons with low back problems, these muscles in particular tend to atrophy. A mere 4.5 pound force is all it takes to collapse an isolated ligamentous spine fixed at the base.[91] The stability of the lumbar spine depends on two muscle systems: the extrinsic stabilizers, which are all the muscles surrounding it, and the intrinsic stabilizers, which are the ligaments and intra-abdominal pressures. The aims of physical therapy to improve these two systems, thereby stabilizing the spine are: (A) Strengthening the abdominal muscles, (B) Strengthening the back extensor muscles, and (C) Strengthening the iliopsoas group. Strengthening the abdominal muscles not only strengthens the extrinsic stabilizers, it also increases the integrity of the intrinsic stabilizers, namely intra-abdominal pressure, which also opposes and thereby minimizes the forces on the lumbar spine. Strengthening the iliopsoas group also strengthens the extrinsic stabilizers. The fact that these muscles weaken in patients with low back pain indicates the necessity for this procedure.[92]

Strength, or power training, involves the use of high forces for short periods of time and primarily affects the fast-twitch fibers (Type II). It has no effect on muscle hyperplasia (increased number of muscle fibers) but does effect hypertrophy of the muscle.[93] Other effects include increased activity of myokinase, which helps maintain a high ATP/ADP ratio.

With strength training, muscles become stronger and larger. Eccentric exercises can produce exertion-induced damage such as changes in the sarcoplasmic reticulum, disruption of cell membranes and changes in the structure of the sarcomeres. Delayed-onset muscle soreness (DOMS) and swelling 24-72 hours after exercise is due to disruption of the muscle-cell membrane allowing proteins such as creatine, kinas and histamine, found in the extracellular environment, to stimulate nociceptors.[94]

Increasing endurance

Muscle training to increase endurance consists of repeated contractions at low levels of force. Such training affects the slow twitch fibers (Type I), which then increase in size, thereby increasing the number of mitochondria. This brings about a higher concentration of oxidative enzymes and increased blood flow.[95] Endurance training can also transform type II fibers. Aerobic endurance training increases the oxidative capabilities of skeletal muscles and might even aid in the prevention of low back pain. The best indicator of aerobic fitness is maximum oxygen consumption (V02 max).

Increasing Range of Motion

Once pain and muscle spasms have been successfully addressed using the techniques described above, then increasing the range of motion is not a problem. But if the pain and spasms are not taken care of, then trying to increase range of motion is an exercise in futility.

Range of motion exercises are introduced as soon as pain and muscle spasms are no longer an issue for the patient. This author does not attempt to passively stretch any structures. As pain and spasms diminish, and with the ever increasing use of isotonic strengthening exercises for the abdominals and back extensors, the patient's range of motion automatically improves. The use of machines to develop strength and endurance also enhances range. One caution: this author avoids and vociferously warns against stretching the hamstring muscles in low back pain patients. As Kapandji points out, forced elevation of the leg with the knee extended can exert a traction force on the nerve roots of as much as 3kg.[96] Since these nerve roots have a resistance to traction of 3.2kg, a trapped root or one shortened by a prolapsed disc could make rough manipulation of the leg liable to rupture axons, resulting in paralysis, usually short-lived but sometimes persisting a long time. For this reason, the senior author never forces stretching of the hip extensors.

The Lasegue sign, for this reason, must always be elicited gently and as soon as the patient feels pain, the therapist must stop. The sign must never be elicited with the patient anesthetized and the pain reflex absent.

The senior author uses other techniques such as contracting-relaxing of the knee extensors, which is more effective than stretching the hamstrings of low back patients.[97]

SPINAL STENOSIS AND DISC DEGENERATION (OA)

Verbiest defined this condition as involving any narrowing of the spinal canal, tunnels of the intervertebral foramen or nerve root canals.[98] Porter et al. clearly demonstrated that persons with small spinal canals are more susceptible than others to backache."
The usual pathologic changes attributed to disc degeneration occur in the intervertebral joint, with the natural healing process

of osteophyte formation, also called spondylosis, or osteoarthritis (OA). The peak of the degeneration process and back pain is during the ages of 30-50 years, and symptoms tend to subside thereafter.

In the lumbar spine, the osteoarthritis changes are primarily in the facet joints associated with intervertebral disc and soft tissue structures cause narrowing of the spinal canal. He called this "triple joint-complex" the cause of spinal stenosis. But whether the narrowing of the spinal canal is degenerative, congenital or developmental, the end result is still called spinal stenosis.

The main problem with the intervertebral joint is narrowing of the disc space with the end result of central stenosis, or foramina entrapment. This gives rise to subluxation of the facet joints. The facets can sublux in the frontal, sagittal and axial planes, leading to joint erosion, recurrent joint effusion and osteophyte formation.

Subluxations of the facet joints, particularly in rotation, can severely narrow the spinal canal. Other consequences of subluxations of the facet joints and narrowing of the disc include shortening, and thus thickening, of the ligament flavum, which further narrows the neural canal. In short, degeneration of the disc and facet leads to canal or lateral stenosis.

When a disc bulges posteriorly, its height decreases and the facet collapses, overrides and hypertrophies. The ligament flavum thickens and buckles, hence instability develops.

Pathophysiology of spinal stenosis, a function of aging, proceeds from mechanical compression of the nerve root to mechanical instability and nerve root ischemia, causing venous stasis and hypertension. The narrowing of the discal space is the main cause of central stenosis, or foramina entrapment in the intervertebral joint. Its prevalence among older patients is not known. An understanding of the pathophysiology of spinal stenosis depends on an appreciation of the interbody joint and two facet joints. The entrapment of the nerve root as a consequence of the narrowing of the disc space and facet joint subluxation manifests as chronic intermittent back pain, resulting from minor irritation due to OA of the facet joints.

History

The most common manifestation is no disabling backache for a number of years in patients over 50 years of age. The major symptom of spinal stenosis of the lumbar region is neurogenic claudication, with aching pain and with or without tingling and numbness (paresthesia) in the buttock or the posterior thigh or calf. The symptom is exacerbated during walking or sometimes on assuming an erect posture or even on extension. Patients ambulate with flexed hips and knees, which helps them to walk greater distances than otherwise possible.

According to Turner et al.,[100] symptoms are eight times more apt to be bilateral in men than in women; unilateral claudication is three times more apt to occur in men than in women. Patients complain of discomfort chiefly in the calves but also in the thighs and feet on walking.

Many patients with degenerative discs and degenerative disease of the facet joints (OA) have no symptoms at all. Some may complain of mild symptoms and still others may have radiating pain down the leg, making it difficult to walk. They complain of reduced flexibility in the lumbar spine, with extension causing the greatest discomfort or dull, aching pain. The main complaint is morning stiffness which resolves as the day goes on and the simian ambulatory stance mentioned above. Patients may be asymptomatic when at rest, but complain of pain in the calves when walking short distances. After resting for a few minutes, they are able to walk again. As the degenerative process continues, they complain of pseudo-claudication, the symptoms of spinal stenosis. These patients also complain of pain when walking downhill, and find relief in positions that flex the lumbar spine, such as bicycling. Their relief in the bicycling position differentiates them from patients with intermittent claudicating due to peripheral vascular disease.

A few patients, it must be remembered, have leg pain only. They complain also of weakness in both lower extremities, numbness and tingling. All flexion activities, such as cycling, bring relief of pain, and extension activities such as walking down an incline or going down stairs cause pain.

According to Porter et al.,[101] patients with back pain have smaller spinal canals than those without back pain. Disc degeneration and the various pathological changes in intervertebral joints such as spondylosis, or ossteophyte formation, lead to stiffening and healing of this joint.

Patients who are 30-50 years of age when back pain peaks usually improve as they age. The process is eloquently described by Kirkaldy-Willis et al.[102]

Except for the minority of patients whose symptoms of spinal stenosis develop when they are over the age of 60 years, most patients can be advised that their symptoms will improve as they get older.

Examination

To the physical therapist, analysis of the patient's gait is of paramount importance. These patients' posture shows a slight flexion of the hips with knees extended, and when asked to ambulate, the flexed hips and knees are exaggerated in the typical simian stance. Range of motion is limited in extension, but flexion is fairly normal. In later stages of the disease, with more degeneration, muscle atrophy, weakness and even asymmetric reflexes may be present. Straight leg raising is usually normal except in a few cases of spinal stenosis with a disc herniation. After the initial neurologic examination, the patient is asked to walk until his symptoms recur, or 300 feet.

Differential Diagnosis

From the history alone, it is often difficult to distinguish the intermittent claudication of neurogenic disease from that of peripheral vascular disease. The following may help to differentiate them:

(1) The bicycle test. Cycling precipitates an attack in those with vascular claudication, but not for those with neurogenic claudication.

(2) Somatosensory potentials after walking.[103]

(3) Pain referred from the lower lumbar region into the thigh and buttocks can mimic neurogenic claudication when the symptoms are due to walking. But patients with spinal stenosis complain of the symptoms with activities other than walking.

(4) Root pathology may sometimes worsen with walking, but spinal stenosis patients may also complain of pain at rest.

Besides peripheral vascular disease, facet joint syndrome also must be differentiated from low back pain with lumbar spine extension. Facet joint syndrome involves referred pain to the leg with extension and ipsilateral side bending. During the early stages, the pain is localized over a single facet joint; then as time goes on, patients complain of pain on rotation and/or extension of the spine with side bending. Many studies, however, question not only the efficacy of treatment, but even the existence of a clinical entity called the Facet Joint Syndrome.[104, 105, 106]

Pathophysiology

A small canal, as mentioned, is only one factor in spinal stenosis. Other factors can be bony or soft tissue elements impinging on the neural structures at the spinal canal or neuroforamen. The degenerative processes seen in spinal stenosis include formation of osteophytes of the vertebral-body end plates, hypertrophy and bony proliferation of the facet joints, and hypertrophy of the anterior facet capsules and of the ligamentum flava.

Verbiest defines spinal stenosis as any condition involving any type of narrowing of the spinal canal, nerve root canals or tunnels of the intervertebral foramina.[107]

The classification system for spinal stenosis developed by Arnoldi et al. is followed herein:[108]

A. Congenital
B. Acquired:
   1. Degenerative
   2. Combined Congenital and Degenerative
   3. Iatrogenic (postsurgical)
   4. Post-traumatic

The following symptoms, alone or in combination, occur in all types of spinal stenosis:

a) Mechanical nerve-root compression, causing radiculopathy,
b) Mechanical instability,
c) Nerve root ischemia,
d) Venous stasis/hypertension.

All these symptoms lead to chronic cauda equina syndrome, and intermittent neurogenic claudication, in addition to pain and weakness of the lower extremities.

Lumbar spinal stenosis (LSS) manifests as low back pain and pain in the lower extremities. The cause is compression of the cauda equina, which may be congenital, degenerative, or both, and leads to stenosis of the lumbar spinal canal and intervertebral foramen. Some authors speculate that the neurogenic claudication may be due to local ischemia of the lumbar nerve roots, brought about by limited blood flow.[109] Impaired motor conduction also has been seen in patients with LSS.[110]

Newer studies describe impaired perception of lumbar position in patients with LSS.[111] These authors point out clinical implications and also include that LSS patients show paraspinal muscle denervation and an abnormal flexion/extension activation.[111]

Differences in Spinal Stenosis and Disc Herniation Symptoms

Patients with spinal stenosis will clinically show symptoms of pain in low back when standing and extending the spine.

Treatment: Unfortunately, controlled, randomized studies of surgical versus non-surgical treatments are wanting. Deyo in his study of patients discharged from the state of Washington during the years of 1986 to 1988, found 18,122 hospitalizations for surgery of the lumbar spine, and out of this number, 3,380 (18.6%) had spinal stenosis.[112] The mean age at surgery in this study is 65 years.

Taylor et al. found a dramatic increase in surgical rates for spinal stenosis during the period from 1979-1981; surgeries increased from 4.0 per 100,000 in 1979-1981 to 7.7 in 1988-1990.[113]

There are significant differences in patients with spinal

stenosis and disc herniations. In patients with spinal stenosis, clinically the symptoms are elicited by standing with extension, and are relieved by standing with flexion or by sitting. On the other hand, with patients who are diagnosed as having disc herniations, their symptoms are clinically elicited by standing with flexion or by sitting. The patterns of epidural pressure and disc pressure are the cause of these differences. In different postures the disc pressure and epidural pressure varies, as shown by Takahashi[1M]; it has been shown that the disc pressure was increased, and the epidural pressure was decreased, by sitting as compared with the respective pressures during upright standing. During lumbar flexion, on the other hand, the epidural pressure is decreased and the disc pressure is increased. This explains the difference in symptoms in different postures for patients with spinal stenosis and disc herniations.

The dearth of prospective or randomized studies of treatment techniques makes it difficult to reach reliable conclusions regarding the natural history of spinal stenosis. In one of the better studies to date, Johnsson et al. described the outcomes of 44 patients treated with surgical decompression and 19 others treated conservatively.[115] Neurophysiologic changes proceeded in all patients; surgery failed to slow the process. The authors concluded that non-surgical treatment yielded good results in one third to one half of cases with only 10% deterioration during the 2-3 year follow-up period. In an earlier study, Tile et al. concluded that aggressive non-surgical measures (therapeutic exercises and epidural shots) were very effective for spinal stenosis patients.[116] They studied 52 patients for 2-8 years and found that 33 (69%) had no difficulty walking, but for 25 patients (48%), standing for long periods was a problem. None of the patients had neurological problems that were exacerbated. Porter argues in favor of a conservative approach because patients with neurogenic claudication tend to reach a plateau of disability and then deteriorate no further.[117] They rarely develop serious paraparesis of the feet and can always walk a short distance. Although surgery often dramatically relieves the symptoms, a conservative approach is reasonable.

Another group of experts, Borenstein, Wiesel and Boden, describe OA and spinal stenosis patients as having a relapsing course with recurrent episodes of back pain that responds to physical therapy. They conclude that surgical intervention is unnecessary. Their 4-year prospective study of spinal stenosis indicates that conservative measures effectively decrease or control symptoms.[118]

Other studies also show the efficacy of conservative management. In a study by Onel from 1984 to 1988, 145 patients were hospitalized for LSS and studied for one month.[119] They were given daily treatments of calcitonin followed by ultrasound and flexion-extension exercises with excellent results:

- pain reduction 91% — significance level .001,
- flexion improved 40% — significance of .001,
- SLR gain 70% — significantly better,
- resumption of usual activities — significantly better,
- global effects 90%,
- greater walking distance 89%.

A 10-year prospective study by Amundsen et al. reached interesting conclusions regarding treatment of LSS by surgical versus conservative means.[120] Over half the conservatively treated patients experienced a satisfactory resolution of their problems. Of the severely afflicted patients, four fifths of those treated surgically experienced a good outcome. "Intolerable" pain was almost always the reason for undergoing surgery. The authors considered the important elements of treatment to be bed rest at the outset, use of an orthosis, attendance at a back school, physiotherapy (consisting of general training and changing to a slightly forward-bending back position) and encouragement early on to resume work and normal activities. The patients in the conservatively treated group wore the same kind of extension orthosis worn by those in the surgically treated group to stabilize the back after surgery. But this device, the authors indicate, may be contraindicated for patients who have problems with extension; extension of the back decreases the volume of the dural sac, increasing compression on nerve and vascular structures, according to several published reports. The outcome might have been different if patients in the conservatively treated group had not worn the orthosis.

Borenstein, Weisel and Boden reported on 32 patients who received no therapy; symptoms lessened in 15% of men, remained unchanged in 70% and worsened in 15%. None experienced severe deterioration requiring surgery during the period of the study.[121]

Goals of treatment

Once the diagnosis is confirmed by clinical examination and MRI or CT, aggressive physical therapy can begin to achieve the following goals: (1) Reduce pain, (2) Increase range of motion, (3) Increase strength and endurance, (4) Increase walking ability and distance, and (5) Resume usual daily activities.

Pain reduction is most important, as it is disabling for most patients. Those with severe pain and stiffness due to OA of the facet joints along with spinal stenosis may be helped by ultrasound treatment. Short-wave diathermy is another acceptable modality for the purpose. This clinician uses interferential therapy and/or low level laser therapy for pain reduction.[122, 123, 124]

Relative rest and restricted activities accompany the medications prescribed by the patient's physician in the protocol which this senior author aggressively pursues. Patients are given a list of "do and do not's" regarding daily activities and their appropriateness for their condition. The choice of therapeutic modality depends on whether the patient's pain is due to OA or to a herniated disc. If the main problem of stenosis is due to OA of the facet joints, the preferable modality is ultrasound to the facet joints involved. If the stenosis is mainly due to a herniated disc, this author uses interferential therapy as described under treatment of discs.

These modalities are followed by traction. This author uses the Cortrell technique. If back pain is the only symptom, then the 90/90 position to unload the spine is used for 30 minutes daily. If radiculopathy is present, this position is used with distraction to ease the compression, thereby relieving the paresthesia.

Strengthening exercises for both the flexors and extensors are begun in non weight-bearing positions, first isometrically, then progressing to isotonically within the patient's pain tolerance. A recent study indicates that patients with LSS show denervation and abnormal activation of lumbar paraspinal muscles. They also appear to have selective type 2 muscle denervation, paradoxically good lumbar endurance and an abnormal flexion-extension cycle in lumbar spinal stenosis.[125]

Cardiovascular training also is advised in addition to strengthening exercises. At our center, we use stationary bicycles as well to strengthen the extensors of the lower extremities. Patients are taught deep breathing and Jacobson's relaxation exercises. They are advised also to take up aquatic exercises or walking in the pool on a daily basis.

Electrical stimulation of the peripheral nerves inhibits pain pathways at the spinal cord level. This key aspect of Melzack and Wall's spinal-gate-control theory was confirmed in Hanai's study: afferent fiber input inhibits C fiber-evoked activity. Hanai considers electrical stimulation of the peripheral nerves to be appropriate and markedly effective, even in cases of chronic back pain, radicular pain, pain of entrapment neuropathy, injured peripheral nerves and spinal injuries.[126]

SPONDYLOLISTHESIS/SPONDYLOLYSIS

Spondylolisthesis (Greek spondylos "vertebra" and olisthesis, "to slip"), the forward slipping of L5 on S1, is due to a major part of the weight of the trunk resting atop the unstable fifth lumbar vertebral body. Certain developmental factors such as trauma, repetitive activities or a particular posture could cause stress fracture of the pars intercularis. Other congenital factors such as lack of integrity of the posterior structures or intrinsic weakness of the bone, as in osteogenesis imperfecta also could cause this problem; in a large series of patients, the defect appeared 95% of the time at the L5 level.[127] It is interesting to note that a large majority of persons with spondylolisthesis go through life with no problems related to this disorder, yet a few individuals with only a minimal degree of slippage complain of severe pain.

Spondylolisthesis has several causes according to the early work of Neughebauer, with which Newman agrees.[128] Their classification has evolved over the last two decades:

(Type 1) Dysplastic. A lack of superior sacral facets or arch of L5, which would halt the forward slipping of L5 on S1.
(Type 2) Isthmic. The typical defect in the pars interarticularis (spondylolysis), allowing L5 to slip forward. This type is

further subdivided.

(Type 3) Degenerative. Disc degeneration or facet degeneration allowing forward slipping of the vertebra.

(Type 4) Traumatic. Acute fractures in the pedicle, lamina or facets, allowing the slipping, but not in the pars.

(Type 5) Pathologic. Paget's disease, for example.

(Type 6) Postsurgical. Forward slipping due to loss of posterior elements secondary to surgical decompression.

Etiology is unknown in the majority of cases. Hardly any cases of spondylolisthesis or spondylolysis have been noted at birth and any caused by trauma are unknown or vague. Child and adult spondylolisthesis differ in natural history, symptom complex and response to treatment.

Spondylolysis occurs chiefly in 6% of the population and at ages 5-7 years. It occurs in about 5% of those over 7 years of age, the group in which it is most frequently seen. As a rule, spondylolysis begins in children past the walking stage and rarely before the age of 5 years.[129, 130] Thereafter the incidence of spondylolysis and spondylolisthesis continues to rise until the age of 20 years, then it remains constant, the same as for the general population.[130] A hereditary component is suggested in spondylolysis with a 29-69% incidence among close relatives, compared to a 4-8% incidence in the general population. However, it is never seen in patients under 5 years of age.

That the onset of symptoms coincides with the adolescent growth spurt is generally agreed and some authors believe that spondylolysis is related to the growth spurt.[131, 132] Others believe that trauma, usually minor trauma, is the cause.[133] Wiltse has done much work on the problem and considers stress or fatigue fracture of the pars intercularis to be responsible for the symptoms.[134] Chronic stress can cause gradual disruption of the pars intercularis or its acute traumatic fracture. Some experts believe that athletes, because of their chronic stresses, have a fourfold increase in incidence of spondylolysis compared to the general population.[135] Female gymnasts are 11% more likely to have spondylolysis than are the rest of the general population.[136] Weight lifters and college football linemen also have an increased incidence. Pars defects are twice as high in men as in women, while spondylolisthesis is seen more often in women.

Flexion movements of the trunk cause shear forces on the lumbar facets and disc spaces. Stress on the pars is greatest when the spine is extended. When it flexes laterally, as in back-walkover in gymnastics, additional forces are added.[136] Severe stress forces concentrate first at the inferior portion of the pedicle, then as the stress is increased, at the pars. Over time, this severe stress causes pars failure.[137]

Clinical history

Pain usually prompts the adult patient to seek medical advice. Child patients are usually brought to medical attention because of poor posture or abnormal gait and if they complain of pain, it is usually localized to the low back. Their symptoms generally coincide with a growth spurt, as previously mentioned. In both children and adults, the pain is aggravated by activity and relieved by rest.

When radicular pain is a complaint, it is due to an irritated nerve, and spondylolisthesis is usually the cause, if this is the case, pain is usually in the posterior thigh due to the involvement of the first sacral root, since most often the slippage takes place at L5-S1. Spondylolysis is most apt to slip into spondylolisthesis between the ages of 9 and 13 years; thereafter, the risk is diminished.[138]

Back complaints are usually not apparent until the age of 35 years, and precipitated by a sudden twisting or lifting movement that brings about an acute episode of leg and back pain. On testing, the patient complains of pain on flexion and relief on extension.[139] Yet certain studies indicate that flexion exercises are more effective than extension in treating patients with spondylolisthesis.[140, 141]

Hamstring tightness is characteristic of both spondylolysis and spondylolisthesis and is seen in children and adults alike. It is the cause of the simian stance, the flexed hips and knees and the backward pelvis tilt that obliterates the lumbar lordosis. In children, the hamstring tightness gives rise to a peculiar gait which P.H. Newman dubbed a "pelvic waddle".[142] This gait is a stiff-legged, short stride that rotates the pelvis forward with each step. Because of this peculiar stride, the patients prefer to run or jog rather than walk. When they do walk, they prefer to keep their knees bent and walk on their toes.

Our understanding of the way disorders of the lumbar spine affect movement is limited at the present time because, as McGregor et al. points out, research studies frequently fail to differentiate between the various disorders and treat all low back pain patients as a whole.[143] We applaud these investigators and we could not agree more when they suggest that in spondylolisthesis, the grade of slip and the type, whether isthmic, traumatic or degenerative, affects global motion parameters. Spinal hypermobility tends to accompany the condition when it entails a defect only and no slip, while hypomobility tends to accompany an actual slip.[143] This distinction is crucial for identifying the condition so it can be treated appropriately. In their study, patients presenting with spondylolysis had greater range of motion in flexion and extension than did those with spondylolisthesis. Those with isthmic spondylolisthesis tended, if

130

the defect was at L5-S1, to have restricted range of motion in extension.[143] These authors clearly make the point that low back patients must not all be treated alike; to do so exposes them to great harm. The diagnosis must determine the therapy.

Physical Examination. Patients complain of a chronic, dull aching pain and cramping along the belt line. Hyperextension and/or rotation exacerbates the pain, as do the repetitive motions involved in sports, gymnastics, wrestling, weight lifting, and fast bowling in cricket.

Patients present with a lumbar lordosis. Viewed from the front, the lower abdomen is thrust forward. In grade I or grade II spondylolisthesis, physical findings are normal along with mild spondylolysis, but flexion may be limited due to tight hamstrings. Viewed from behind, a depression or palpable step-off may appear over the 5th lumbar spinous process. The majority of patients who are symptomatic have a lumbar scoliotic list which is not structural and disappears on prone tying.[144]

Children with spondylolysis or spondylolisthesis have tight hamstrings; in the straight leg raising (SLR) test, the therapist can usually lift the leg only a few inches off the examination table before causing pain. In normal children, 70-80 degrees of hip flexion are usual. Some authorities believe the muscle is tight because an irritated nerve root causes it to spasm. Others link the tight muscle as a mechanism to stabilize the L5-S1 joint.[144]

To sum up, the important findings on examination are: (1) pain on extension. The symptom is exacerbated when the patient stands on one leg and attempts to extend the spine. (2) Paraspinal muscle spasm and tight hamstrings with SLR of few degrees.

Radiological diagnosis is chiefly made using plain X-rays. On AP, oblique and lateral views show a defect in the pars. Oblique view (figure) shows a line resembling the collar of a Scottish terrier. See Figure 14.

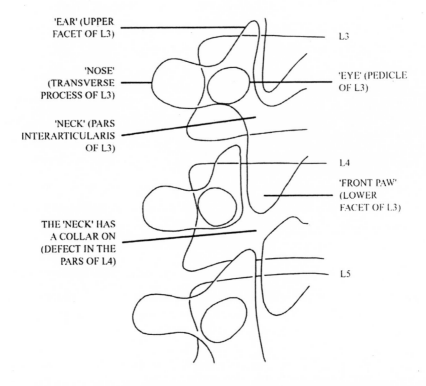

Diagram to illustrate the fracture and the 'collar of the Scottie dog'.

Figure 14

Bone-scan with single-photon emission computed tomography (SPECT) is *the* gold standard of radiological diagnosis. MRI is used when a disc degeneration is suspected along with spondylolysis.

Natural History of Spondylolysis and Spondylolisthesis

A unilateral pars defect is not associated with further slip or disability and subjects with bilateral L5 pars defect have a clinical course similar to that of the general population.[145] Their

45-year follow-up study indicates the progression of the slip slows markedly up to age 50 years, and none of the subjects reached a 49% slip. They advise parents of children with a lumbar pars lesion or low-grade spondylolisthesis to expect a benign course for the first 50 years. They further advise that there is no reason for children with spondylolysis and low-grade spondylolisthesis not to compete in sports.

Acute spondylolysis usually occurs at the lower lumbar levels, but may occur at any level. The pain of spondylolysis is a combination of discogenic and spondylolysis pain, i.e. pain arising from sensory, slow conducting pain fibers of C type in the spondylolysis tissue.[146] Nordstrom et al. explain defective healing seen on the pars: the sparsity of stromal innervation in spondylolysis accounts for the lack of neurogenic bone-regulating mechanisms.[146]

Whether or not spondylolisthesis progresses significantly depends upon the individual's pelvic anatomy. When the standing posture increases shear stress at the L5 junction and posterior element dysplasia coexistents, the ability to resist such shear stress may be significantly reduced, creating an environment conducive to progression of the spondylolisthesis.[147]

Treatment

In the acute phase, rest with activity is indicated, as with all back conditions. Exercises are begun when the patient's muscle spasms and pain have abated.

The Goals of Physical Therapy are:
1. reduce pain
2. increase range of motion
3. increase strength and endurance
4. resume former daily activities, working and playing

sports.

To rest the fracture and allow healing of isthmic spondylolysis in adolescents, anti-lordotic Boston braces and corsets help limit activity for a period of six to nine months until the patient is pain-free. Until then, care must be taken to manage the pain. Medication must accompany physical therapy. We use interferential therapy, low level laser therapy, or ultrasound, for pain as well as for muscle spasms. All three modalities also have a healing, osteoblastic effect on fractures. We also show patients a back-school film teaching them the "do's and do not's" for their condition.

We teach pain-free flexibility exercises to be done while the patient is wearing the brace with the spine in a neutral position in flexion; this relieves stress on the posterior elements, thereby minimizing pain. The exercises are increased after the patient is out of the brace, still keeping within the pain-free range. This author never passively stretches hamstrings, but uses contracting/relaxing or PNF techniques to safely achieve the same purpose.

Strengthening exercises can begin as soon as the patient is out of the brace, and preferably is pain-free. The exercises are to tighten abdominal muscles, back extensors, quadratus lumborum, glutei and all other muscles in the lower extremities, in order to stabilize the lumbar spine and keep the intradiscal pressures low. Exercises must be performed on an unmovable, stable surface, as an unstable one could harm the patient. This therapist avoids isotonic extension exercises, but uses isometric back exercises within pain-free limits. These patients are best treated cautiously and carefully guarded, as are young athletes. For instance, if they resume sports and pain recurs, they must go back to the anti-lordotic brace and be treated until pain and spasms subside completely.[148]

As with other back problems, the purpose of the exercises is to strengthen muscles and increase intra-abdominal pressure so as to strengthen muscles and increase abdominal pressure, which in turn stabilizes the lumbar spine. For this purpose, co-contraction exercises are unnecessary and this author questions the entire rationale of such.

For these patients, this author does not recommend extension exercises either, unless they are performed isometrically. The only supporting evidence available at present is a study by Sinaki et al. in which, after three years, 62% of patients given flexion exercises improved while none of those given extension exercises showed any improvement.[149] Their conclusions favor the treatment program at our clinic.

A young athlete with less than 25% slip, muscle spasms and low back pain must not be allowed vigorous activity until symptoms abate. Sometimes these patients are given an antilordotic brace. If, despite rest and wearing a brace, the pain and spasms do not abate, they are advised to take up a less strenuous sport, because additional injury could be permanently disabling.

If the slip is Grade II, i.e., more than 50%, the patient is apt to present with exaggerated lordosis, hamstring tightness and a waddling gait. Again, a less strenuous sport is recommended. If conservative care does not resolve the patients' symptoms, a posterolateral fusion is recommended.

Patients with symptoms of a Grade III slip or more, with nerve root involvement, require surgical intervention, decompression and fusion.[150]

DEGENERATIVE DISC DISEASE (SPONDYLOSIS)

Degenerative disc disease, an aging process of the lumbar spine, takes place mainly in the disc and facet joints and manifests late in the third decade of life. It is diagnosed radiologically, but prior biochemical and histological processes are evident.

The first change to occur in the disc is the decrease in water content in the nucleus pulposus, making the disc less shock-absorbent. Then changes in the collagen in the annulus fibrosis lead to tearing in the lamella. Besides the loss of water in the nucleus, proteoglycan also is lost and collagen is increased. In addition to changes in the disc, the vertebral body also undergoes change, hence the three-joint complex is involved. Stresses and strains cause the vertebral body to form osteophytes, which can be seen on X-rays. The ligamentum flavum becomes hypertrophic, causing nerve irritation.

The L4 disc undergoes extensive destructive changes not seen in any other musculoskeletal tissue. This disc consists of a nucleus pulposus composed of a gelatinous mass in juveniles, with an annulus fibrosus composed of collagen fibers arranged in lamellae formation and cartilaginous end plates separating these structures from adjacent vertebral bodies. Many clinicians believe that the L4 disc is a main source of pain, but whether the destructive changes are due to aging or other degenerative processes is difficult to determine.[151] According to Norbert Boos, a decrease in blood vessels in the end plate is destructive to the integrity of the disc matrix.[152] These authors believe that the resulting poor nutrition of the disc leads to its degeneration. In addition, with skeletal maturity, the exit routes are closed with the closing of the epiphysis in the vertebral bodies, so that large molecules cannot diffuse out of the nucleus pulposus. These authors point out that the poor nutrition, decline in proteoglycan organization and concentration, loss of cell synthesis and density, and the greater degrading enzyme activity relative to matrix synthesizing activity, all may contribute to disc degeneration.

Other studies indicate that inflammatory reactions in the disc and nerve roots cause back and leg pain.[153]

Despite severe disc changes seen on MRI, the majority of subjects are asymptomatic.[154] Some animal studies show a pressure-dependent pump action that helps in fluid exchange back and forth across the disc boundary.[155] Weight-bearing leads to fluid output which lowers volume and reduces nutritional activity, leading to changes in disc tissue, mainly remodeling of the tissue, and depending on the amount and duration of axial loading, to disc degeneration.[155] Increasing duration of loads clearly leads to more pronounced degeneration, with clefts and fissures appearing in histological preparations in the annulus fibrosus and with additional herniation of discal material and osteophyte formation.[156] Another important finding: discs loaded with five times the body weight showed morphologic changes after 14 to 28 days compared to unloaded discs. Therefore, therapeutic intervention should begin early in the degenerative process to maintain tissue integrity or stimulate its repair.[156]

In clinical practice, diagnosis is by radiological demonstration of the disc height and osteophyte formation.[157] For macroscopic grading of disc degeneration we follow Nachemson's system:

(Grade I) the nucleus pulposus is gelatinous, shiny and easily separated from the annulus,

(Grade II) the nucleus pulposus is somewhat more fibrous but still clearly defined from the annulus,

(Grade III) macroscopic changes appear in both the nucleus pulposus and the annulus with some blurring of the boundary between them,

(Grade IV) marginal ostephytes appear in the vertebral bodies, severe macroscopic changes, with fissuring and cavitation, appear in both the nucleus and the annulus.

Demographics

Discs degenerate during the second decade of life in men, earlier than in women. Onset of low back pain peaks between ages 25-30 years and sciatica at about 27 years when, as Andersson clearly demonstrates, 40% of all discs, male and female, show Grade II degeneration and 10% of male discs show Grade III.[157]

Interestingly, fifteen years may pass before the onset of disc protrusion with radiating pain. In a study by Miller, A. A. et al., 90% of discs they autopsied were Grade II; of the male discs, 30% were Grade III, 10% Grade IV, while only 20% of female discs were Grade III and none were Grade IV.[158] The authors concluded that men subject their discs to greater axial loading than women do, and also that longer avascular nutritional pathways in men cause them more severe and earlier disc degeneration. Although 90% of specimens showed signs of disc degeneration on X-ray, only 37% had a history of back disorders.

Miller et al. found that in upright postures, the disc at L3 is horizontal but the disc at L5-Sl is inclined between 20 and 65 degrees, which increases shear forces at that level by 36-217% over those at the L3 level where they are zero. Although they relate the high shear loading to the high incidence of spondylolysism, spondylolisthesis, and even disc herniations at this level, the authors do not consider it a cause of disc degeneration, which they feel could lessen the risk of disc protrusion.[158]

History

Some patients present with morning stiffness and pain that abates with movement as the day progresses. Most subjects do not complain of pain, despite radiological evidence, but a few seek medical advice. Of these, most are in their late thirties or early forties.

Persons in certain occupations are particularly vulnerable to disc disease: truck drivers, pilots, tractor drivers— those exposed to vibrations and those whose jobs require repetitive bending and twisting. Smoking and riding in a car for long periods also increase the risk of disc disease. Riding in a car, aside from the vibration, may exacerbate pain because of prolonged sitting.

Pain radiating down the lower extremities or paresthesis that intensifies with certain movements can be used to pinpoint the location of the particular problematic structure in the three-joint complex. Increased symptoms on flexion are due to involvement of an anterior element such as a desiccated disc or a herniated disc. Extension causes pain that cannot be directly related to posterior structures, but sometimes the facet joints are involved.

Physical Examination

As with all patients, the modified Kraus-Weber test is used. As a rule, the physical examination is unremarkable except that range of motion is limited. Flexion is limited by pain of a desiccated disc or a herniated disc. Extension is limited due to facet joint problems. On palpation, spasms of the paravertebral muscles are felt. Depending on whether the anterior or the posterior structures are involved, the patient shows either an exaggerated lordosis or obliteration of the lumbar lordosis. X-rays, CT scans and MRI studies are used to confirm the diagnosis. EMG studies help to locate the positions of nerve impingement if disease is present at many levels.

Treatment

Patients must be educated about their problem and informed that although degenerative disc disease is irreversible, treatment can relieve the symptoms and retard the degenerative process. Treatment can also improve the quality of life by easing and facilitating performance of normal daily activities.

Pain management is foremost in the treatment protocol; if radicular pain is a complaint, Cortrell traction can be used for the pain. Thereafter only the 90/90 position is used to unload the spine, which reduces intradiscal pressure.[159] White and Punjabi believe that the 90/90 position benefits most low back pain patients because the supine position reduces discal pressure, the straight back minimizes posterior disc bulging, and flexed hips and knees eliminate tension in the psoas muscle so that the disc pressure and stretch on the sciatic nerve is minimal.[160] In addition, reduced axial loading aids in the nutrition of the disc, as mentioned. The senior author has used this technique for many years with excellent results. After spending 30 minutes in this position in the clinic, patients are advised to continue the program at home — twice daily for 30 minutes if they are in severe pain and once daily otherwise.

Strengthening exercises help stabilize the lumbar spine, first isometric, later adding isotonic, always within the patient's pain-free range. Flexibility exercises for all muscles of the extremities and the lumbar spine, exercises to increase range of motion and cardiovascular exercises are also incorporated into the program.

Lumbar Flexion Injuries

Floyd and Silver[161] proved that in complete spinal flexion, the erector spinae muscles are totally relaxed (electrical silence on EMG), a condition termed the flexion-relaxation response. In this position, then, the ligamentous structures must maintain the integrity of the spine. Working in this position, Floyd and Silver warn, can lead to injuries of the intervertebral discs. Ligamental and annular stresses associated with lumbar flexion make this a position that no one, whether a patient or a normally healthy individual, should assume.[161] No one disputes this. Some controversy exists, however, regarding what motion actually takes place during flexion. Most authorities cite the lumbo-pelvic rhythm in which the first 60 degrees of flexion take place in the lumbar spine and flexion beyond this takes place in the hips. See Figure 15.

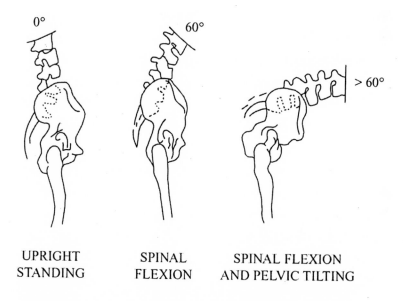

| UPRIGHT STANDING | SPINAL FLEXION | SPINAL FLEXION AND PELVIC TILTING |

The lumbo-pelvic rhythm is the textbook description of how people bend over. The first 60° takes place in the lumbar spine (flexing), while further rotation of the torso is accomplished with rotation about the hip. We have never measured this sequence in anyone - from professional athlete to back patient.

Figure 15

Olympic weight lifters, however, do the opposite; that is, they lock the lumbar spine in a nearly neutral position and flex only at the hips. McGill maintains that this is prophylactic; it is therapeutic for patients to avoid the stresses of lumbar flexion in this way. McGill observes that the term flexion-relaxation is inappropriate because relaxation of the extensor muscles seems only to occur in an electrical sense.[162] During fall spinal flexion, these muscles stretch, generating a substantial amount of elastic force.

PIRIFORMIS SYNDROME

The piriformis muscle can be implicated in sciatica-like symptoms when the hip is externally rotated. The muscle originates from the pelvic surface of the 2nd, 3rd and 4th sacral vertebrae. It inserts into the upper border and greater trochanter of the femur. Since the sciatic nerve root (L4-S3) lies under the piriformis muscle and above the obturator internus muscle, an injury to the piriformis muscle can cause it to contract, thereby compressing the sciatic nerve against the obturator internus muscle. It may sometimes cause pain over the path of the sciatic nerve, all the way to the leg and foot; without a specific dermatome, the symptoms are a foot drop with a limp. This is not a true sciatica but a "pseudosciatica." The differential diagnosis with a true sciatica is that the SLR is negative with this syndrome, and the muscles above the piriformis, such as the gluteal and tensor fascia latae, will be spared and EMG studies will be normal for these muscles while the muscles below the piriformis will show denervation activity.

The test for the piriformis syndrome is the Freiburg's test, i.e. pain with internal rotation of the hip. The piriformis muscle is an external rotator of the hip, and internally rotating the hip will stretch this muscle, causing spasm and reflex pain. The other test is pain on resisted external rotation and abduction of the hip.

Epidemiology

There is no particular group at risk.

Treatment

Mainly non-steroid anti-inflammatory drugs, followed by physical therapy such as a piriformis stretch exercise program. Bed rest when indicated, followed by cold packs and modalities like ultrasound or interferential therapy for pain management.

The pain, called pseudosciatica, travels down the sciatic nerve to the foot, but not in a dermatomal pattern. The disorder is not commonly seen and can be difficult to diagnose. Over a period of more than four decades intimately involved with low back pain, this senior author has seen no more than ten patients with piriformis syndrome. See Figure 16.

Evaluation

In one diagnostic test, the Freiburg test, internal rotation of the hip reproduces the pain. Since the piriformis is a lateral rotator of the hip, internal rotation stretches the muscle with resulting reflex spasm and pain.

Another test is external rotation of the hip and abduction with resistance; this demonstrates weakness and pain.

Care must be taken to differentiate this syndrome from disorders that cause inflammation of the sacroiliac joints, which can irritate the origin of the piriformis and cause pain down the sciatic nerve.

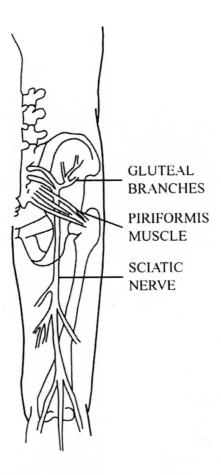

GLUTEAL
BRANCHES

PIRIFORMIS
MUSCLE

SCIATIC
NERVE

Piriformis syndrome. The priformis muscle originates from the sacrum and inserts on the medial side of the greater trochanter of the femur. Spasm of the priformis muscle will affect motor and sensory supply to the lower extremity but will spare the proximal gluteal muscles.

Figure 16

PERIPHERAL VASCULAR DISEASE

Patients with peripheral vascular disease complain of claudication, which affects muscle groups rather than dermatomes. Circulatory problems with diminished peripheral pulses rather than sensory problems are the cause.

CHAPTER 5 NOTES

1. Kelgren JH. On the distribution of pain arising from deep somatic structures with charts of segmental pain areas. *Clinical Science.* 1939; 4: 35.
2. Steindler A, et al. Differential diagnosis of pain low in the back: allocation of the source of pain by the procain hydrochloride method. *Journal of the American Medical Association.* 1938; 110: 106-112.
3. Nordin, M. 2000 Presidential address to the international society for the study of the lumbar spine. *Spine.* 2001; 26: 851-856.
4. Waddell, G. Point of View. *Spine.* 1996; 21: 2898.
5. Spitzer WO, LeBlanc FE, Dupuis M, et al. Scientific approach to the assessment and management of activity-related spinal disorders. *Spine.* 1987; 12: 1-55.
6. Wiesel SW, Feffer HL, Borenstein DG. Evaluation and outcome of low back pain of unknown etiology. *Spine.* 1988; 13: 679-680.
7. Finch, P. Spinal pain- an Australian perspective. In McGill, S. *Law Back Disorders.* Champaigne, EL: Human Kinetics; 1999: 7.
8. Thompson EN. Back Pain: Bankrupt expertise and new directions. *Journal of Pain Research Management.* 1997; 2: 195-196.
9. McGill S. *Law Back Disorders.* Champaign, IL: Human

Kinetics; 2002: 7.

10. Dillane JB, Fry J, Kalton G. Acute back syndrome: study from general practice. *British Medical Journal.* 1966; 3: 82.

11. Braggins S. *Back Care: a Clinical Approach.* New York: Churchill Livingstone; 2000.

12. Troupe JD, Martin JW, Lloyd DC et al. Back pain in industry: a prospective study. *Spine.* 1981; 6: 61-69.

13. Styf JR. Pressure in the erector spinae muscle during exercise. *Spine.* 1987; 12: 675-679.

14. Almikinders, L.C., Garrett, W.E. Jr.et al. m: Malone T, Duncan P, William G, eds., *Muscle Injury and Rehabilitation.* New York: Williams & Wilkins; 1988.

15. McCully KK, Faulkner JA. Injury to skeletal muscle fibers of mice following lengthening contractions. *J Appl Physiol.* 1985; 59: 119-126.

16. Jesper L, Peter Schjerling, Bengt Saltin et al.; Muscles, Genes and Athletic Performance. *Scientific American.* 2000. Sept: 48-55.

17. Howell JN, Chlenoun G, Conaster R. Muscle stiffness, strength loss, swelling and soreness following exercise induced injury in humans. *Journal of Physiology.* 1993; 464; 183-196.

18. Cooper, R.G. Understanding paraspinal muscle dysfunction in low back pain: a way forward. *Annals of Rheumatic Disease.* 1993; 52: 413.

19. Nikolaou PK, MacDonald BL, Glisson RR, Seaber AV, Garrett Jr. WE. Biomechanical and histological evaluation of muscle after controlled strain injury. *American Journal of Sports Medicine.* 1987; 15: 9-14.

20. Borenstein, DG, Wiesel SW, Boden SD. *Low Back Pain.* 2nd ed. Philadelphia: W.B. Saunders Company; 1995: 322.

21. Cooper RG. Understanding paraspinal muscle dysfunction in

low back pain: a way forward. *Annals of Rheumatic Disease.* 1993; 52: 413.

22. Gordon GH, Johnson EW, Laban MM. The fibrositis syndrome. Archives of Physical Medicine Rehabilitation, In: Frymoyer JW, Gordon S, eds. *New Perspectives on Low Back Pain.* Park Ridge, IL: American Academy of Orthopedic Surgeons; 1988: 366-367.

23. Fernando CK. Diagnosis, prognosis, and treatment strategies for peripheral nerve injuries and sciatic scoliosis due to active disc herniations. *Biofeedback Foundation of Europe;* 2003.

24. Travell J, Rinzler S, Herman M. Pain and durability of the shoulder and the arm. In Frymoyer JW, Gordon S, eds. *New Perspectives on Low Back Pain.* Park Ridge, IL: American Academy of Orthopedic Surgeons; 1988: 366-367.

25. Roland, M.D. A critical review of the evidence for a pain-spasm-pain cycle in spinal disorders. In Frymoyer JW, Gordon S, eds. *New Perspectives on Law Back Pain.* Park Ridge, IL: American Academy of Orthopedic Surgeons; 1988: 366-367.

26. Pedersen et al. Reported in: Lactic Acid- The Latest Performance-Enhancing Drug, *Science.* 2004; 305: 1112-1113.

27. Nielsen OB, et al. *Journal of Physiology.* 2001. Reported in: Lactic Acid- The Latest Performance-Enhancing Drug. *Science.* 2004; 305: 1112-1113.

28. Chaffin DB. Localized muscle fatigue: Definition and measurement. *Journal of Occupational Medicine.* 1973; 15: 346-354.

29. Holding DH. Fatigue, m: Hockey R, ed. *Stress and Fatigue in Human Performance.* New York : John Wiley & Sons; 1983 : 145-165.

30. Bates BT, Ostemig LR, James SL. Fatigue effects in running.

Journal of Motor Behavior. 1977; 9: 203-207.

31. Bauwens, P. The "multifidus triangle" syndrome as a cause of recurrent low back pain. *British Medical Journal.* 1955; 2: 1306.

32. Elliot A, McMaster DH. The biomechanical properties of tendon strength in relation to muscular strength. In: *Clinics in Sports Medicine.* Vol. 2. W.B. Saunders Company: Philadelphia; 1983: 73.

33. Kellgren JH. In: *New Perspectives on Law Back Pain.* Park Ridge, EL: American Academy of Orthopedic Surgeons; 1988.

34. Simons DG, Travell J. Myofascial origins of low back pain. *Clinical Science.* 1982; 73:81-88.

35. Waddell G. Point of view. *Spine.* 1996; 21: 2898.

36. Simons DG. Fibrositis/Fibromyalgia: a form of myofascial trigger points? *Postgraduate Medicine.* 1982; 23: 81-88.

37. Bernard TN Jr., Kirkaldy-Willis WH. Recognizing specific characteristics of nonspecific low back pain. *Clinic of Orthopedics.* 1987; 217: 266-280.

38. Carr D, Gibertson L, Frymoyer J, et al. Lumbar paraspinal compartment syndrome: a case report with physiologic and anatomic studies. *Spine.* 1985; 10: 816-820.

39. Styf JR. Pressure in the erector spinal muscle during exercise. *Spine.* 1987; 12: 675-679.

40. Fardon DF. Nomenclature and classification of lumbar disc pathology. *Spine.* 2001; 26: 461-462.

41. Fernando, C.K. Treatment of low back pain; review of recent research findings with rationale and technique of treatment. *Proceedings of the Seventh International Congress of the World Confederation for Physical Therapy.* London: World Confederation for Physical Therapy; 1974: 313.

42. Frymoyer J, Gordon S. *New perspectives on Low Back Pain.*

Park Ridge, IL: American Academy of Orthopedic Surgeons; 1988: 362-367.

43. Borenstein DG, Wiesel SW, Boden SD. (1995). *Low Back Pain.* 2nd ed. Philadelphia: WB Saunders Company; 1995:186-192

44. Horwitz T. Lesions of the intervertebral disc and ligamentum flavem of the lumbar vertebrae: an anatomic study of seventy five human cadavers. *Surgery.* 1939; 6: 410.

45. Salminen JJ, Erkintalo J, Pentti A, Oksanen A, Kormano MJ. Recurrent low back pain and early disc degeneration in the young. *Spine.* 1999; 24: 1316-1321.

46. Weber H. Lumbar disc herniation: a controlled perspective study with ten years of observation. *Spine.* 1983; 8: 131-140.

47. Saal JA, Saal JS. Non-operative treatment of herniated lumbar intervertebral disc with radiculopathy: An outcome study. *Spine.* 1989; 14: 431-437.

48. Nachemson AL. The lumbar spine: an orthopedic challenge. *Spine.* 1976; 1: 59.

49. Kelsey JL, Ostfield AM. Demographic characteristics of people with acute herniated lumbar intervertebral discs. *Journal of Chronic Disease.* 1975; 28: 37-50.

50. Estridge MN, Rouhe SA, Johnson NG. The femoral nerve stretching test: a valuable sign in diagnosing upper lumbar disc herniation. *Journal of Neurosurgery* 1996:57:813-817.

51. Dyck P. The femoral nerve traction test with lumbar disc protrusions. *Surgical Neurosurgery.* 1976; 6: 163-167

52. Kirkaldy-Willis WH. The relationship of structural pathology to the nerve root. *Spine.* 1984; 9: 49-52.

53. Moore RJ. Origin and fate of herniated lumbar intervertebral disk tissue. *Spine.* 1996; 21: 2149-2155.

54. Adams MA, Hutton WC. Prolapsed intervertebral disk: a hyperflexion injury. *Spine.* 1982; 7: 184-191.

55. Vernon, R. et al. Degenerative changes in the intervertebral disks of the lumbar spine and their sequlae. *Rheumatology Rehabilitation, 6,* 13-21.

56. Adams, M.A., & Hutton, W.C. Prolapsed intervertebral disk: a hyperflexion injury. *Spine, 7,* 184-191.

57. Brickmann, P. Laboratory model of lumbar disk protrusion- Fissure and fragment. *Spine.* 1994; 19: 228-235.

58. Lu YM, Hutton WC, Gharpuray VM. Do bending, twisting and diurnal fluid changes in the disc affect the propensity to prolapse? A visco-elastic finite element model. *Spine.* 1996; 21: 2570-2579.

59. Matusai H. Significance of sciatic scoliotic list in operated patients with lumbar disc herniation. *Spine.* 1998; 23: 338- 342.

60. Arangio GA. Significance of lumbosacral list and low back pain: a controlled radiographic study. *Spine.* 1990; 15: 208- 210.

61. Porter RW. Back pain and trunk list. *Spine.* 1986; 11: 596- 600.

62. McKenzie RA. Manual correction of sciatic scoliosis. *New Zealand Medical Journal.* 1976; 76: 194-199.

63. Porter RW. Back pain and trunk list. *Spine.* 1986; 11: 596- 600.

64. Porter RW. Back pain and trunk list. *Spine.* 1986; 11: 597- 599.

65. Porter RW. Back pain and trunk list. *Spine.* 1986; 11: 596- 600.

66. Porter RW. Back pain and trunk list. *Spine.* 1986; 11: 596- 600.

67. Porter RW. Back pain and trunk list. *Spine.* 1986; 11: 596- 600.

68. Porter RW. Back pain and trunk list. *Spine.* 1986; 11: 596-

600.

69. Matsuai H, Ohmori K, Kanamori M, Ishihara H, Tsuji H. Significance of sciatic scoliotic list in operated patients with lumbar disc herniation. *Spine.* 1998; 23: 338-342.

70. Matsuai H, Ohmori K, Kanamori M, Ishihara H, Tsuji H. Significance of sciatic scoliotic list in operated patients with lumbar disc herniation. *Spine.* 1998; 23: 338-342.

71. Matsuai H, Ohmori K, Kanamori M, Ishihara H, Tsuji H. Significance of sciatic scoliotic list in operated patients with lumbar disc herniation. *Spine.* 1998; 23: 338-342.

72. Hirayama J, Takahashi Y, Nakayima Y, Takakashi K, Yamagata M, Moriya H. Effects of electrical stimulation of the sciatic nerve on background electromyography and static stretch reflex activity of the trunk muscles in rats: possible implications of neuronal mechanisms in the development of sciatic scoliosis. *Spine.* 2001; 6: 602-609.

73. Hirayama J, Takahashi Y, Nakayima Y, Takakashi K, Yamagata M, Moriya H. Effects of electrical stimulation of the sciatic nerve on background electromyography and static stretch reflex activity of the trunk muscles in rats: possible implications of neuronal mechanisms in the development of sciatic scoliosis. *Spine.* 2001; 6: 602-609.

74. Ambrose C, Scott A, Ambrose A, Talbot EO. Chronic low back pain: assessment using surface eleotromyography. *J of Occup and Environ Med.* 2000; 42: 660-669.

75. Conor W, Kurgansky ME, Derby R, Ryan DP. Disc stimulation and patterns of referred pain. *Spine.* 2002; 27: 2776-2781.

76. Conor W, Kurgansky ME, Derby R, Ryan DP. Disc stimulation and patterns of referred pain. *Spine.* 2002; 27: 2776-2781.

77. Anderson GBJ, Deyo RA. Sensitivity, specificity, and

predictive value: a general issue in screening for disease and in the interpretation of diagnostic studies in spinal disorders. In: Frymoyer JW, Gordon S, eds. *The Adult Spine: Principles and Practice.* 2nd ed. Philadelphia: Lippincott-Raven; 1997: 305-317.

78. Delitto A, Erhard RE, Bowling RW. A treatment-based classification approach to low back syndrome: identifying and staging patients for conservative treatment. *Physical therapy.* 1995; 75: 470-489.

79. Bigos SJ, Bowyer 0, Braen G, et al. Acute low back problems in adults. Clinical Practice Guidelines No. 14. *AHCPR Publication, No 95 - 0642.* Rockville MD: Agency for Health Care Policy and Research; 1994.

80. Dyck P. Femoral nerve traction test with lumbar disk protrusions. *Surgical Neurology.* 1976; 6: 163-167.

81. Shiqing X, Quanzhi Z, Dehao F, Anhui H. Significance of the straight leg raising test in the diagnosis and clinical evaluation of lower lumbar intervertebral-disc protrusion. *Journal of Bone Joint Surgery.* 1987; 69A: 517.

82. Gunn CC, Chir B, Milbrat *WE.* Tenderness at motor points: a diagnostic and prognostic aid to low back injury. *Journal of Bone Joint Surgery.* 1996; 58: 815.

83. Deyo RA, Diehl AK. Rosenthal M. How many days of bed rest for acute low back pain? A randomized clinical trial. *New England Journal of Medicine.* 1986; 315: 1064-1070.

84. Rozenberg S, Delval C, Rezvani Y, et al. Bed rest or normal activity for patients with acute low back pain. *Spine.* 2002; 27: 1487-1493.

85. Merskey M, et al. *Classification of Chronic Pain Syndromes and Definition of Pain Terms.* 2nd ed. Seattle: IASP; 1994.

86. Finneson BE. *Law Back Pain.* 2nd ed. Philadelphia, PA: Lippincott Co; 1984

87. Fernando, CK. Letter to the Editor. *Physical Therapy.* 1991; 71: 167.

88. Cottrell GW. The treatment of low back pain. *Orthopedic Trans.* 1981; 1: 80.

89. Nachemson A. Lumbar intradiscal pressure. *Acta Orthop Scand.* 1960; 43 (suppi): 1-104

90. Rozenberg S, Delval C, Rezvani Y, et al. Bed rest or normal activity for patients with acute low back pain. *Spine.* 2002; 27: 1487-1493.

91. Morris JM. Role of the trunk in the stability of the spine. *Journal of Bone and Joint Surgery.* 1961; 43A: No. 3.

92. Fernando, CK. Treatment of low back pain; review of recent research findings with rationale and technique of treatment. *Proceedings of the Seventh International Congress of the World Confederation for Physical Therapy.* Chicago IL: Forest Hills Back Institute; 1974: 310.

93. Adams MA, Bogduk N, Burton K, Dolan P. *Biomechanics of Back Pain.* Edinburgh: Churchill Livingstone; 1995:53.

94. Adams MA, Bogduk N, Burton K, Dolan P. *Biomechanics of Back Pain.* Edinburgh: Churchill Livingstone; 1995:53.

95. Adams MA, Bogduk N, Burton K, Dolan P. *Biomechanics of Back Pain.* Edinburgh: Churchill Livingstone; 1995:53.

96. Kapandji IA. *The Physiology of the Joints.* 2nd ed. Edinburgh: Churchill Livingstone; 1974: 127.

97. Fernando, CK. Treatment of low back pain; review of recent research findings with rationale and technique of treatment. *Proceedings of the Seventh International Congress of the World Confederation for Physical Therapy.* London: World Confederation for Physical Therapy; 1974.

98. Verbiest H. Results of surgical treatment of idiopathic developmental stenosis of the lumbar vertebral canal: a review of twenty-seven years' experience. J Bone Joint Surg

Br 1977. 59:181-188.

99. Porter RW. The spinal canal in symptomatic lumbar disc disease. *Journal of Bone Joint Surgery.* 1996; 60B: 2046-2052.

100. Turner JA, Ersek M, Herron L, et al. Surgery for lumbar spinal stenosis. Attempted meta-analysis of the literature. *Spine.* 1992; 17:1-8.

101. Porter RW. Spinal canal in symptomatic lumbar disc disease. *Journal of Bone Joint Surgery.* 1996; 60B: 2046-2052.

102. Kirkaldy-Willis WH et al. Pathology and pathogenesis of lumbar spondylosis and stenosis. *Spine.* 1978; 3: 319-328.

103. Keim HA, Hajdu M, Gonzalez E, Brand L, Balasubramanian E. Somatosensory evoked potentials as an aid in the diagnosis and intra-operative management of spinal stenosis. *Spine.* 1985; 10: 338.

104. Moran R, O'Connell D, Walsh MG. The diagnostic value of facet joint injections. *Spine.* 1988; 13: 1407.

105. Jackson RP, Jacobs RR, Montesano PX. Facet joint interjection in low back pain: A prospective statistical study. *Spine.* 1988; 13: 966.

106. Jackson RP. The facet syndrome: myth or reality? *Clinical Orthopedics.* 1992; 279:110.

107. Verbiest H. Further experiences on the pathological influence of a developmental narrowness of the bony lumbar vertical canal. *Journal of Bone Joint Surgery.* 1955; 37B: 576-583.

108. Arnoldi CC, Brodsky AE, Cauchoix J et al. Lumbar spinal stenosis and nerve root entrapment syndrome: definition and classification. *Clinical Orthopedics.* 1976; 115

109. Porter RW. Spinal stenosis and neutrogenic claudication. *Spine.* 1996; 21: 2046-2052.

110. Kondo M, Matsuda H, Kureya S, Shimazu A. Electrophysiological studies of intermittent claudicating in lumbar stenosis. *Spine.* 1989; 14: 862-866.

111. Leionen V, Maatta S, Taimela S, Hemo A, Partanen J, Kansanen M. Impaired lumbar position sense in association with postural stability and motor and somatosensory- evoked potential findings in lumbar spinal stenosis. *Spine.* 2002; 27: 975-983.

112. Deyo RA. Morbidity and mortality in association with operations on the lumbar spine. The influence of age, diagnosis, and procedure. *Journal of Bone Joint Surgery.* 1992; 74A: 536-543.

113. Taylor V. Low back pain hospitalizations: Recent United States trends and regional variations. *Spine.* 1994; 19:1207-1213.

114. Takashaki K. Changes in epidural pressure during walking in patients with lumbar spinal stenosis. *Spine.* 1995; 20: 2746-2749

115. Johnsson KE, Uden A, Rosen I. The effect of decompression on the natural course of spinal stenosis: a comparison of surgically treated patients and untreated patients. *Spine.* 1991; 16: 615-619.

116. Tile M. Spinal stenosis: results of treatment. *Clinical Orthopedics.* 1976; 115: 104-108.

117. Porter RW. Spinal stenosis and neutrogena claudicating. *Spine.* 1996; 21: 2046-2052.

118. Borenstein DG, Wiesel SW, Boden SD. *Low Back Pain.* 2nd ed. Philadelphia: WB Saunders; 1995:206.

119. Onel D, Sari H, Donmez C. Lumbar spinal stenosis: Clinical radiologic and therapeutic evaluation in 145 patients: conservative treatment or surgical intervention? *Spine.* 1993; 18: 291-298.

120. Amundsen T, Weber H, Lilleas F, et al. Lumbar spinal stenosis: clinical and radiologic features. *Spine.* 1995; 20: 105-185.

121. Borenstein DG, Wiesel SW, Boden SD. *Low Back Pain.* 2nd ed. Philadelphia: *WB,* Saunders; 1995: 206.

122. Johnson M, et al. Investigation into the analgesic effects of interferential currents and transcutaneous electrical nerve stimulation and experimentally induced ischemic pain in otherwise pain-free volunteers. *Physical Therapy.* 2003; 83: 208-223.

123. Nwuga VC. Ultrasound in treatment of back pain resulting from prolapsed intervertebral disc. *Archive of Physical Medicine Rehabilitation.* 1983; 64: 88-89.

124. Scarcova J. Influence of ultrasound galvanic currents and short wave diathermy on pain intensity with osteoarthritis. *Spine.* 2003; 28: 324-331.

125. Leionen V. Paraspinal muscle denervation, paradoxically good lumbar endurance and abnormal flexion-extension cycle in lumbar spinal stenosis. *Spine.* 2003; 28: 324-331.

126. Hanai F. Nerve electrical stimulation for pain. *Spine.* 2000; 25: 1890-1892.

127. Lowe RW. Standing roentograms in spondylolisthesis. *Clinical Orthopedics.* 1976; 117:80-84.

128. Newman PH. Etiology of spondylolisthesis. *Journal of Bone Joint Surgery.* 1963; 45B: 39-59.

129. Rowe GG, Roche *MB.* The etiology of separate neural arch. *Journal of Bone Joint Surgery.* 1953; 35A: 102-109.

130. Wiltse LL. Spondylolisthesis in children. *Clinical Orthopedics.* 1961; 21: 156-163. 131-Barash HL. Spondylolisthesis and tight hamstrings. *Journal of Bone Joint Surgery.* 1970; 52A: 1319-1328.

131. Dandy DJ. Lumbosacral subluxation (Group I

spondylolisthesis). *Journal of Bone Joint Surgery.* 1971; 53B: 578-595.

132. Turner RH, Bianco A.J. Jr. Spondylolysis and spondylolisthesis in children and teenagers. *Journal of Bone Joint Surgery.* 1971; 53A: 1298-1306.

133. Wiltse LL, Widell EH, Jackson DW. Fatigue fracture: The basic lesion in isthmus spondylolisthesis. *Journal of Bone Joint Surgery.* 1975; 57A: 17-22.

134. Jackson DW, Wiltse LL, Cirincione RJ. Spondylolysis in the female gymnast. *Clinical Orthopedics.* 1976; 117: 68-73.

135. Rothman RH, Simeon FA. *The Spine.* 2nd ed. Philadelphia: WB Saunders; 1982: 264-268.

136. Farfan HF. Mechanical etiology of spondylolysis and spondylolisthesis. *Clinical Orthopedics.* 1976; 117: 40-55.

137. Wiltse LL, Widell EH, Jackson DW. Fatigue fracture: The basic lesion in isthmus spondylolisthesis. *Journal of Bone Joint Surgery.* 1975; 57A: 17-22.

138. Borenstein DG, Wiesel SW, Boden SD. *Law Back Pain.* 2nd ed. Philadelphia: WB Saunders; 1995:208.

139. Borenstein DG, Wiesel SW, Boden SD. *Low Back Pain.* 2nd ed. Philadelphia: WB Saunders; 1995:211.

140. Sinaki M. Lumbar spondylolisthesis, retrospective comparison and three year follow-up of two conservative treatment programs. *Archive of Physical Medicine Rehabilitation. 1989; 70: 594.*

141. Newman PH. A clinical syndrome associated with severe lumbosacral subluxation. *Journal of Bone Joint Surgery.* 1965; 47B: 472-481.

142. McGregor AH, Cattermole HR, Hughes SPF. Global spinal motion in subjects with lumbar spondylolysis and spondylolisthesis: Does the grade or type of slip affect global spinal motion? *Spine.* 2001; 26: 282-286.

143. Rothman RH, Simeon FA. *The Spine.* 2nd ed. Philadelphia: WB Saunders; 1982: 267-269.

144. Beutler WJ, Fredrickson BE, Murfland A, Sweeney CA, Grant WD, Baker D. Natural history of spondylolysis and spondylolisthesis. *Spine.* 2003; 28:1027-1035.

145. Nordstrom D. Symptomatic lumbar spondylolysis: Neuroimmunologic studies. *Spine.* 1994; **19:** 2752-2758.

146. Lukasz J. Radiographic markers in spondyloptosis. *Spine.* 2002; 27: 2021-2025.

147. Micheli L. Use of modified Boston brace for back injuries in athletes. *Sports Medicine.* 1980; 8: 351-356.

148. Sinaki M. Lumbar spondylolisthesis: Retrospective comparison and three-year follow up of two conservative treatment programs. *Archive of Physical Medicine Rehabilitation.* 1989; 70: 594.

149. Cole AJ, Herring SA. *Low Back Pain Handbook.* Philadelphia: Hanley & Belfus, Inc; 2003: 105-108.

150. Vernon-Roberts B. Age related and degenerative pathology of intervertebral discs and apophysial joints, In: Jayson MIV, ed. *Lumbar Spine and Back Pain.* Edinburgh: Churchill Livingstone; 2002: 17-41

151. Boos N. Classification of age related changes in lumbar intervertebral disks. *Spine.* 2000; 27:2631-2644.

152. Olmarker K. Inflammatogenic properties of nucleus proposus. *Spine.* 1995; 20: 665-669.

153. Boos, N et al: Natural history of individuals with asymptomatic disk abnormalities in MRI. *Spine.* 2000; 25:1484-1492.

154. Iatridis JC. Compression induced changes in intervertebral disk properties in a rat tail model. *Spine.* 1999; 24: 996-1002.

155. Markus WK. New in-vitro animal model to create

intervertebral disk degeneration and to investigate to the effects of therapeutic strategies to stimulate disk regeneration. *Spine.* 2002; 27: 2684-2690.

156. Andersson GBJ. Roentographic measurement of lumbar intervertebral disk height. *Spine.* 1981; 6: 154-158.

157. Miller AA. Lumbar disc degeneration: Correlation with age, sex and spine level in 600 autopsy specimens. *Spine.* 1988; 13: 173-178.

158. Nachemson AL. Lumbar spine: an orthopedic challenge. *Spine.* 1976; 1: 59.

159. White AA, Punjabi MM. *Clinical Biomechanics of the Spine.* 2nd ed. Philadelphia: Lippincott-Raven; 1990: 424.

160. Floyd WF, Silver PHS. Function of erector spinae in flexion of the trunk. *Lancet.* 1951; 1: 133-134.

161. McGill S. *Law Back Disorders.* Champaign, IL: Human Kinetics; 2002: 92.

VI

CLINICAL EVALUATION

To properly and correctly treat the patient's problems, we must first understand exactly what the problem is. Needless to say, low back pain is a symptom, not a disease. It is important that the patient be carefully evaluated before ANY treatment is undertaken to relieve the pain, since a dangerous medical condition, needing attention, may be present. A definitive diagnosis is the essential guide to proper treatment, which can prevent complaints from becoming chronic, and can minimize unnecessary surgery, which presently occurs in 6-9% of cases. In many of these, if the patient had been competently examined and then given appropriate physical therapy, the result would have been improvement in less than three months, as in most cases treated by physical therapists.

To reach an accurate diagnosis, our clinical evaluation must follow the most reliable, efficient strategies, i.e. the time-tested methods of allopathic medicine. This therapeutic system of western science is accepted the world over.

Despite this, some academics with little knowledge of pathology-based diagnoses and even less of clinical practice, impelled by the need to "publish or perish," devise abbreviated systems that do away with scientific diagnoses. But to short-circuit the diagnostic process for back pain, as a few therapists want to do (Delitto, Fritz, Spitzer, Wemeke),[1-4] serves no useful purpose; on the contrary, it is most dangerous both to patients and to the profession because it puts patients at risk of receiving inappropriate treatment. At present, the challenge is to find better, more efficient ways to treat low back pain, not to abort key elements of the diagnostic process that are considered necessary for all other complaints.

Standards set by the American Physical Therapy Association[5] in its *Guide to Physical Therapy Practice*, with which we agree, call for an anatomic-pathological diagnosis to be made, so that treatments can be focused on impairments and functional limitations. This is in line with approach of the World Health Organization[6] in its *International Classification of Impairments. Disabilities, and Handicaps* (ICIDH), which provides a conceptual framework on which to standardize and monitor disabling and chronic conditions. Impairment is defined as loss of anatomic, physiologic or psychological function or structure, that is, edema or losses of strength, range of motion, sensations, proprioception, etc. A correct diagnosis is the guide to the specific problems and to the type and extent of care indicated. The problems are then treated using physical therapy modalities.

For 94% of patients with low back pain who are referred to physical therapy for treatment, the disorders are of mechanical origin. These mechanical problems form the subject of this book, namely sprains and strains, disc herniations, spinal stenosis, osteoarthritis, spondylolysis/spondylolisthesis and adult scoliosis (for a discussion of which see other textbooks dealing with this subject). These patients can be diagnosed and their losses of anatomical, physiological and psychological functions addressed using physical therapy measures.

White & Punjabi's[7] improvement of the work of Charnley[8]

provides a system for the treatment of these patients. In 1955 Charnley[8] described the mechanisms of I-V disc pathology and correlated the patho-anatomic factors with a clinical presentation and treatment of these multiple conditions seen in patients. The senior author has updated those treatment modalities for his patients using this hypothesis: most patients seen in the clinic do not present themselves with a single patho-anatomic problem, but a multiplicity of problems, hence the difficulty in treating these low back pain patients. One has to keep this in mind prior to diagnosis and evaluation, and the problem becomes compounded when a single patient may have both a muscle and ligamentous strain or sprain with an annular rupture. Therefore, it is both ludicrous and harmful when certain therapists come up with schemes which are single modality treatments diagnosed by a few signs and symptoms rather than the accepted allopathic paradigm. Problems can only be properly addressed when treatments are based on complete, accurate diagnoses. The accepted allopathic paradigm is imperative in such cases. The essential elements include:

1. a carefully-taken history,
2. physical examination and observation, and
3. additional sensitive and specific laboratory and radiological tests such as X-rays, CT scans, EMGs and MRIs as needed to confirm the diagnosis.

HISTORY

The standard, detailed, systematized history is a most powerful tool for reaching a definitive diagnosis of a patient with low back pain. It also gives the therapist insight into the patient's current emotional, social and economic status, all of which can affect pain and recovery. The diagnostic work-up also requires a work sheet and a pain map.

Red Flags

Certain symptoms are red flags to alert the clinician that the patient's problems are beyond the scope of physical therapy and must be referred to an internist interested in back pain. Such symptoms include fever, chills, intractable pain mainly at night, weight loss, night sweats, incontinence, loss of sensation in the perineum or anal regions and progressive muscle weakness.

Important Symptoms

Patients often report include low back pain, reported by 90% and pain radiating distally to one or both legs, reported by about 70-80%.

Other important symptoms that the clinician must look for are neurological problems and spinal deformity, though they are much less common. Occasionally, patients with gastrointestinal, genitourinary, hip or vascular disease have back pain which must be differentiated by means of the history and physical examination. In doubtful cases, the patient must be referred to an internist with expertise in this area for a diagnostic work-up.

Demographic Factors

Age, sex, marital status, race, occupation, leisure and athletic activities and social history may relate to the problem. Young patients are more prone to strains, sprains, discogenic pain and spondylolysis then are older patients, who are more apt to have spinal stenosis, degenerative joint disease and osseous problems such as vertebral fractures. Men are more prone to have ankylosing spondylitis, discogenic pain or strains and sprains due to athletic involvement than are women, who are more apt to have osteoporosis or fibromyalgia.

Certain occupations can cause back pain as well. Workers involved in heavy manual lifting, for example, are prone to mechanical low back pain. Person in stressful occupations with little or no job satisfaction are prone to pain with non-organic components. Whether or not the problem is job-related, the legal aspects must be addressed. If the patient has missed work in the past, the more time missed, the poorer the chances of an early return to work.

Leisure and athletic activities and lifestyle must be included in the history. Smoking, alcohol consumption and obesity are risk factors for low back pain and herniated intervertebral disc.[9]

A complete, carefully taken history must include:

1. The date the pain began.

2. Whether the onset was sudden or gradual.

3. The mechanism of injury.

Note where and how it occurred. Was it a fall at home, an accident at work or during sports? Was it a motor vehicle accident? Was it caused by flexion, as in picking up a dropped pencil or other item? Or was it caused by extension, twisting, coughing, or sneezing?

If related to athletics, what sport and what movement was involved? Sports-related injuries involving flexion and rotation movements, as in golf, baseball and tennis, have a high incidence of sprains/strains and discogenic pain. In sports involving hyper-extension such as gymnastics, rowing and ballet, the injury is apt to be to the facet joints or sprains and strains of extensor muscles.

In work-related injuries, the history must indicate the nature of the accident, its cause, the site of the pain and such legal aspects of the problem as pending litigation, Workman's Compensation, time off and whether recreational activities are limited to the same degree as work-related activities.

4. Location of the pain. The patient is given a map of the body and asked to mark the location of back pain, leg pain, bilateral leg pain, pain below the knees, pain in front of the thigh, etc. The patient is also asked to mark the location of any numbness, tingling, pins and needles, or other sensations. These pain maps are inconclusive by themselves, but can be invaluable in assessing the total picture while reaching a diagnosis.[10]

When the cause is mechanical, back pain localizes to the lumbosacral spine. When the cause is damage to such structures as the facet joints, discs, muscles and ligaments around the lumbar spine, pain is referred to the buttocks, thigh and paraspinal muscles. On the other hand, pain that radiates from the low back down the lower extremity in a dermatomal pattern indicates irritation of nerve roots.

In cases of disc disease, disruption of the annular fibers of the outer lamellae causes low back pain. But if the disc is protruded, intradiscal pressure is lowered so there is no low back pain, unless the protruded disc impinges on a nerve root; this gives rise to radiating pain down the lower extremity.

Referred pain felt below the knee is rare, while pain due to root irritation – known as radiating pain or radicular pain – may be felt on the calf or even on the dorsum of the foot. Pain from compression of the 4th lumbar root usually radiates down the front of the thigh. Some authorities believe that irritation of a nerve root causes parasthesia such as numbness. Parasthesias involving the lateral border of the foot may be due to a problem at S1 and numbness over the dorsum of the foot and big toe may be due to a problem at L5.

Discal pain can cause radiating pain down the leg even at rest, but not in cases of spinal stenosis. With spinal stenosis, the spinal canal is compromised and neural structures are squeezed so that extension activities cause radiating pain down the lower extremities.

Psychogenic pain is not localized as is nerve root pain and does not appear on dermatomal patterns as can be seen on pain diagrams.

5. Quality and quantity of the pain. Is it aching, stabbing, boring, burning, muscular or another kind of pain? Is it constant or intermittent?

6. Pain and activities. It is best to ask the patient specific questions: Does it hurt in the morning when you bend over the wash basin? Can you make the bed? Is the pain worse when you walk or climb stairs? Is the pain made worse by prolonged sitting, standing or walking?

Certain positions and movements increase the pain of mechanical disorders of the lumbar spine. Usually, these disorders improve with rest and are aggravated by movement.

Flexion motions aggravate disc pain. Extension movements aggravate facet pain and pain due to spinal stenosis. Discogenic pain is made worse by maintaining the same posture for a long time. Prolonged sitting with forward flexion raises intradiscal pressure and aggravates disc pain.

Bed rest helps patients with muscle strain; contracting the muscles with resistance causes pain. Passive motions, on the other hand, cause pain in strained ligaments.

A history of pain when standing up from a sitting position or from coughing, sneezing, laughing or exerting pressure during bowel movements is suggestive of root compression.

7. Peripheral symptoms. Arm or leg pain could be focal or diffuse. When a single nerve root is compressed, the paresthesia is in a well-defined anatomic pattern like a dermatome. Diffuse symptoms, on the other hand, indicate that the spinal cord or multiple roots are involved, resulting in a pattern of pain and numbness or weakness in multiple dermatomes.

A herniated nucleus pulposus typically produces a focal radiculopathy, while a central spinal stenosis more often produces a diffuse pain picture with weakness and bilateral numbness.

8. Claudication can be either neurogenic or vascular in origin. Patients with spinal stenosis complain of leg pain in the calf on walking or on standing still. This is due to neurogenic claudication. For relief of their symptoms, they usually sit down. These patients can usually bicycle for a long time or walk uphill with no difficulty because the lumbar spine is flexed during these activities. On the other hand, walking downhill causes severe pain in the calf muscles because the spine is extended during this activity.

In vascular claudication, symptoms are relieved after resting for 1-2 minutes and there are no symptoms on standing still.

9. Medical attention. Did the patient go to an emergency room or hospital? Were X-rays or MRI taken? Were any treatments given?

Conclusion

This history will reveal the cause of pain and weakness, whether a neurological or structural disorder exists, how significant the disorder is and what problems are entailed. With this information, the clinician can generate a working diagnosis.

Radiography, including magnetic resonance imaging (MRI) and electromyography (EMG) can confirm the diagnosis and also help guide the treatment. Without the careful clinical evaluation, however, radiography by itself can lead to incorrect diagnoses and unnecessary treatments such as manipulations and surgery for problems that should be addressed using physical therapy modalities.

For purposes of the history and physical examination, the spinal column can be divided into two parts: 1) the structural part consisting of the vertebrae and joints, and 2) the neurological part consisting of the spinal cord, cauda equina and nerve roots. Symptoms relating to the structural part are axial in nature while those relating to the neurological part are peripheral or radicular in nature.

PHYSICAL EXAMINATION AND OBSERVATION

The physical examination is of paramount importance for the diagnosis of mechanical disorders of the lumbar spine, which includes nearly 90% of low back complaints.[12] By correctly performing physical examination, including tests that are sensitive and specific for the condition, the problem can be diagnosed quickly and accurately. Sensitivity of a test is its ability to indicate the presence of a particular disease or injury, or to denote PID (positive in disease). Specificity of a test is its ability to correctly indicate the absence of a disease, or to denote NIH (negative in health).

Tests that are neither sensitive nor specific for the disease in question are useless. For example, the U.S. National Institute for Occupational Safety and Health (NIOSH)[13] studied tests for low back pain to find a reliable group of well-defined tests for their *Low Back Atlas.* Using reliability as the criterion, they chose nineteen unrepresentative tests. Six of these are various measures of left-right pelvic tilt and another four measure lumbar lordosis. Unfortunately, neither pelvic tilt nor lumbar lordosis is related to low back disability. So these tests, although highly reliable, are not particularly useful, being neither specific nor sensitive for low back pain. The only test for spinal movement is the lateral flexion test. Thus the NIOSH Atlas is of doubtful clinical value.[14]

To be useful, a test must be reproducible, as in the McKenzie technique, intertester reliability is poor for assessments of low back syndrome[15] and does not improve after postgraduate training in the McKenzie system, which is general in many clinics. Furthermore, the McKenzie system makes no mention of sensitivity or specificity of their diagnostic tests, hence we do not advocate their use.

Most of the classification systems used in some clinical areas are inherently weak in many aspects. According to Riddle, the McKenzie System, Delitto System and the Quebec Task Force System are weak in areas of construct validity, reliability, and generalizability. In addition to this, face validity is also a problem with all of these systems.[16]

The Modified Kraus-Weber Evaluation is still the clinical evaluation of choice, based on the original work of Kraus and Weber as modified by this senior author in 1966.[17, 18] The tests have a very high degree of sensitivity and specificity for low back pain and disc herniation. The examination must include the following:

1. **Observe the patient's spine from behind and from the sides with the upper body bare.** Patients are asked to disrobe down to the waist, but women are to retain their halter tops. First, view the spine from behind to see if the iliac crests are in line, then from the sides to view the curvatures of the spine, noting the lumbar lordosis, whether it is normal, exaggerated in hyperlordosis, or flat, obliterated due to pain and muscle spasms. Note any sciatic list, or deviation of the lumbar spine away from the midline. With

sciatic list, note also whether a raised iliac crest may be seen on one side. If the sciatic list disappears on lying prone, it is due to a disc herniation rather than a structural scoliosis, which does not disappear on lying prone. Note any other spinal deformities such as kyphosis, or rounded shoulders. If the kyphosis is fixed, it is certain that the patient is in an advanced stage of ankylosing spondylitis. Spondylolisthesis patients have a quite noticeable L5 spinous process.

2. **Palpate the lumbar spine at this stage,** feeling each spinous process. It is well to keep in mind that if any deformity is noted in flexion, it appears at L5-S1 and L4-L5. In patients with spondylolisthesis, there is a step-deformity in the L5-S1 processes. Pain on the spinous process during palpation is a sign of possible degenerative disc disease. Then palpate the facet joints for tenderness and muscle spasms by feeling 2 cm from the midline on either side. Patients with spondylolisthesis present with flexed knees; their abnormal posture is due to tight hamstrings.

See Figures 17, 18, 19, 20, and 21.

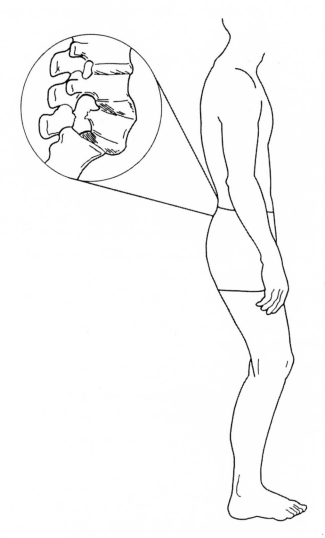

Altered posture due to spondylolisthesis

Figure 17

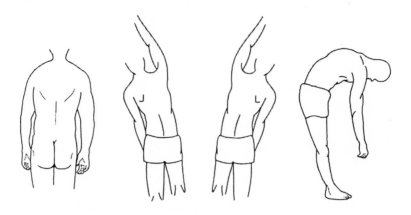

Posterior assessment   Lateral bending   Forward bending

Evaluation of the lumbar spine

Figure 18

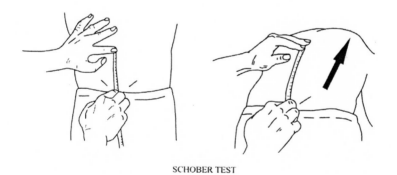

SCHOBER TEST

Figure 19

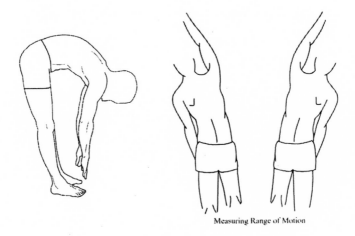

Measuring Range of Motion

Figure 20

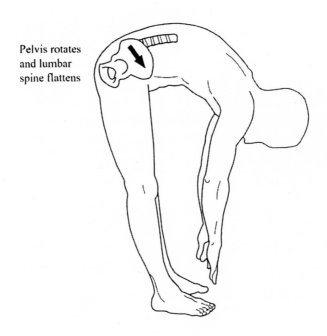

Pelvis rotates
and lumbar
spine flattens

Figure 21

3. **Measure range of motion for flexion.** With the patient standing normally, use a tape measure and record the distance from the patient's fingertips to the floor. Then ask the patient to bend forward without bending the knees and to stop at the point where it becomes painful. Note any rhythm problems during this movement. In a healthy spine, normal lumbar lordosis reverses smoothly during this movement. When the patient bends with the hips, maintaining the lumbar lordosis, it is a sign of back disease.[19] While the patient is in the flexed position, again measure the distance from fingertips to ground. Have the patient extend from the flexion while watching for any rhythm problems or any catch on extension. Note any resulting pain. If the patient is unable to extend without using the hands to crawl up the legs, it is a sign of instability. The normal range for forward flexion is 40-60 degrees, which is equivalent to a distance of 3-6 inches from fingertips to ground at the flexed position. This test by itself has no diagnostic significance, but it can be used to demonstrate functional improvement; in this way, it can be a source of encouragement to the patient.[20]

After undergoing this test, a patient with a sciatic list and a unilateral protective spasm will now have the spine tilted to one side with the iliac crest lowered on that side. Sciatic list, also called lateral shift, or lumbosacral list is seen in only about 5.6% of patients with low back pain — certainly not up to 56% as claimed by McKenzie.[21] McKenzie's treatment for this, a lateral shift maneuver, is not only unnecessary but harmful and erroneous.[22]

Some authorities use the Schober Test to measure flexion on

the lumbar spine itself. To perform this test, mark a point midway over the upper sacrum. Then measure 10 centimeters above this and mark another point here. The distance between these two points increases when the lumbar spine is flexed. In normal subjects, the increase is at least 50%. Patients with discogenic pain will complain of pain and demonstrate limited motion during this test.[23]

4.   **Observe range of motion for extension.** This senior author makes a general estimate of the range, noting whether the patient complains of pain. Then, if the range seems severely limited, he makes a measurement using a goniometer. Normal range is 20-35 degrees. When hyperextension is painful, various causes are possible: narrowed intervertebral foramen impinging on spinal nerves, facet joint apposition or spinal stenosis narrowing the spinal canal and causing pseudo-claudication.

5.   **Examine soft tissue.** Observe tenderness but be aware that agreement between observers is poor for this symptom. Palpate for muscle spasm, though this, too, is unreliable.[24] This senior author studies Surface Electromyography (SEMG) on the erector spinae muscles with the patient lying prone and sitting; specificity and sensitivity are very high and inter-observer agreement is reliable.

6.   **Measure lateral flexion.** The patient is asked to bend sideways, or to slide the hand down the side of the thigh toward the knee, then the distance from the fingertips to the floor is measured. Pain associated with this flexing to the side could be due to stretching muscular or ligamentous structures and not diagnostically significant, but it may be due to articular disease or disc protrusion lateral to the nerve root. For interesting descriptive studies of lateral

flexion and rotation, see Moll.[25]

7. **Check neurological signs.** Inter-observer agreement for the neurological examination as well as for the test, SLR, is very high and within acceptable levels.[26] Waddell's signs are too unreliable to be of significance, as are pain drawings.

8. **Test muscle strength with the patient supine** on the treatment table:

   a) Abdominal muscles and hip flexors. Have the patient keep hands at sides and legs straight while raising the trunk until the scapulae are about 13 inches from the treatment table and holding the position for 10 seconds.

   b) Abdominal muscles alone — crook tying. With the hips at 45 degrees, have the patient sit up with the scapulae 13 inches from the table and hold the position for 10 seconds.

   c) Illiopsoas group alone (eccentric work for the psoas). The therapist positions the patient's hip and knees at 90-100 degrees, then asks the patient to hold the position, as the therapist attempts to extend the hip by pushing on the thighs.

   d) Straight leg raising (SLR). The patient is told to relax, then the therapist lifts the patient's leg, holding it by the ankle until the patient complains of pain. At this point, a goniometer is used to measure the angle of the raised leg with the table, or if the therapist is experienced, the angle can be estimated visually. A rise of 20-40 degrees is positive. Up to 70 degrees can be positive. Pain beyond 70 degrees is due to tight hamstrings.

   e) Crossed SLR. The patient is asked to raise the unaffected leg and if this causes pain in the affected leg, the angle of the raised leg is measured. Pain when the rise is 20-70 degrees is positive.

9. **Test muscle strength with the patient prone,** a pillow under the stomach:

   f) Upper back extensor strength. Patient is asked to lift head and shoulders from the table while keeping hands by the sides. Range of movement is noted, only up to the point of pain.

   g) Lower back extensor strength. The patient is asked to lift the lower limbs one at a time and hold the position for 10 seconds. Again, range of movement is noted, up to the point of pain.

10. **Test weak muscles for nerve root involvement.** Muscles of the lower extremity have dual or triple innervations. The predominant root is in capitals, iliopsoas, LI, L2, L3, adductors, L2, L3, L4, quadriceps, L2, L3, L4, tibialis anterior, L4, L5, extensor hallucis longus, L5, S1, semitendinosis, semimembranosis, L4, L5, S1, S2, peronei, L5, S1, gluteus maximus, L5, S1, S2, and gastrocnemius, S1, S2.

    a) Tibialis anterior. Ask the patient to walk on his heels. Inability to do so indicates weakness of the dorsiflexors of that foot (L4 root involved).

    b) Gastrocnemius. Have the patient rise up on the toes of one foot. Inability to do so indicates weakness of the gastrocnemius muscle (S1 root involved).

    c) Quadriceps. Ask the patient to lie supine on the treatment table, then lift one leg 2 inches from the table, keeping both legs straight. Inability to do so or delayed extension of the knee indicates weakness of the quadriceps muscle (L3-L4 roots involved).

    d) Extensor hallucis longus. The criterion for a differential diagnosis for L5 root lesion is weakness of the extensor hallucis longus, before any weakness of the tibialis anterior (dorsiflexor of ankle, L4 - L5).

e) Flexor hallucis longus. In the case of S1 root involvement, the flexor hallucis longus weakens before any noticeable weakening of the gastrocnemius.

f) Hip abductors. The Trendelenburg's sign indicates weakness of the hip abductors: when the patient stands on one leg, the hip on the unsupported side sags. See Figure 22.

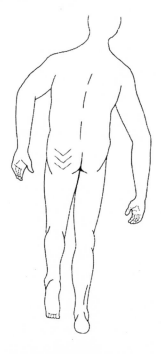

Delayed Trendelenburg test

Figure 22

Some authorities[27] believe that tenderness of certain muscles is a sign of root irritation. Some examples: gastrocnemius soleus complex is tender when S1 root is irritated; anterior tibial muscles are tender when L5 root is irritated; quadriceps muscle is tender when L4 root is irritated.[27]

In examining muscles for weakness, it is advisable to test both sides.

11. **Sensory Examination** must be meticulously performed in order to detect minor changes. Gross changes are easily seen. Ideally, the patient's affected side is compared with the unaffected side using the same number of stimuli, ten pin pricks for example, on each side. Dermatomes are usually well localized, but it must be remembered that dermatomal areas overlap and their distribution varies from one patient to another. Autonomous sensory zones are relatively constant and must be examined.[28]

See Figures 23 and 24.

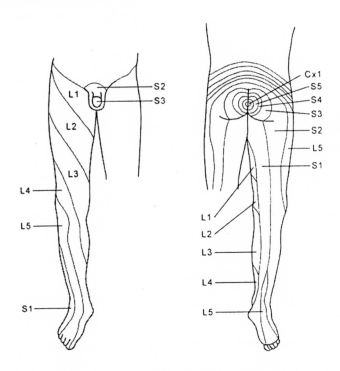

Sensory distribution of lumbar and sacral nerves

Figure 23

180

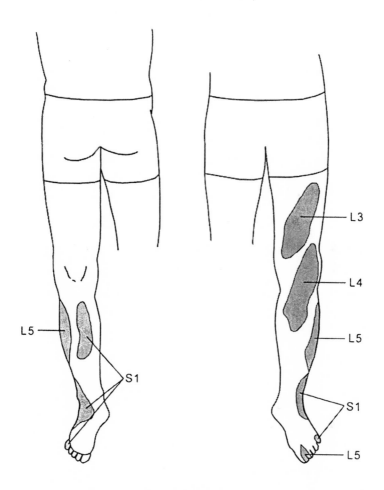

Autonomous sensory zones.

Figure 24

12. **Tests of Root Tension.** These tests stretch peripheral nerves, drawing them over any foreign body such as a herniated disc or osteophyte and reproducing the pain the patient complains of in the affected nerve root. A positive result, therefore, confirms that a herniated disc or an osteophyte is present.

a) *Straight leg raise* (SLR), or Lasegue's sign, is the classic test of nerve root tension. With the patient supine, gradually lift one extended leg. If this movement elicits pain in the same area as paresthesia down the leg in the distribution of the lower lumbar or sacral nerve roots, the sign is positive. Pain and paresthesia in the low back or thigh due to tight hamstrings is not indicative of a root lesion and the sign is negative.

Kapanji terms the pain felt on the posterior aspect of the thigh due to tight hamstrings when the lower limb is extended and nearly vertical as a false positive Lasegue's sign.[29]

When the lower limb is extended with knee straight, the nerve roots freely glide up to 12 mm through the intervertebral foramen.[28] In the presence of a large osteophyte, or more commonly, a prolapsed disc, the nerve must stretch over a longer distance and thus causes pain. The sciatic nerve reaches its maximum tension at up to 60 degrees flexion, and beyond that the pain is diagnostically irrelevant. However, the degree of flexion that causes pain, 10, 20 or 30 degrees, quantifies the severity of the prolapsed disc or the osteophyte.

Caution is essential whenever performing the SLR test. Never stretch the tight hamstrings of a patient with low back pain. An ever-present danger exists, if a herniated disc is present, of rupturing axons, and this could result in paresis (incomplete loss of power) or paralysis of the innervated muscles. As soon as pain is noted, stop the maneuver. See Figures 25, 26, 27, 28 and 29.

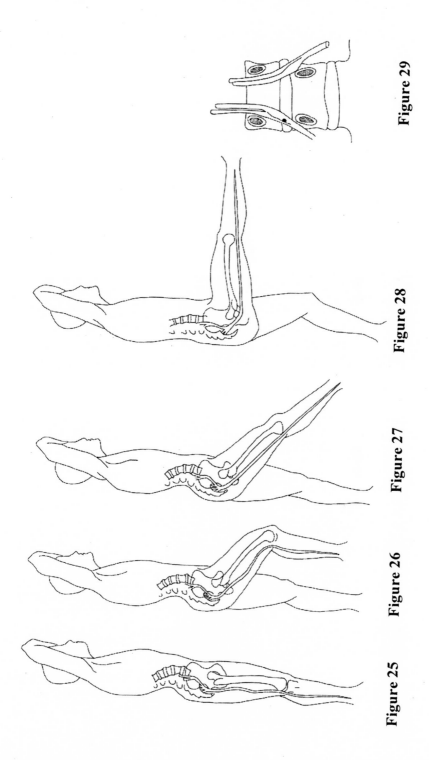

Figure 25

Figure 26

Figure 27

Figure 28

Figure 29

In Fajersztajn's[30] modification of the SLR test, dorsiflexion is added if the patient feels pain while the extended leg is being raised. If this increases pain, the test is positive. See Figures 30 and 31.

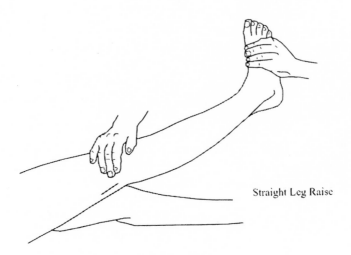

Straight Leg Raise

Figure 30

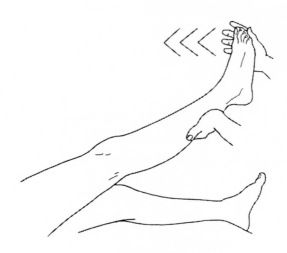

Foot dorsiflexion test

Figure 31

b) Crossed SLR. When the SLR test performed on the patient's affected leg reproduces pain and paresthesia in the unaffected leg, the test is positive. This confirms compression of a nerve due to a herniated nucleus pulposus, possibly by sequestration.

c) Femoral nerve stretch test. With the patient lying prone, gradually flex the knee, then extend the hip. If pain and paresthesia are produced in the anterior thigh, the test is positive for lesions of L3 and L4 roots.

d) Ely's test. Care must be taken not to confuse this test with the femoral nerve stretch test. Ely's test demonstrates a contraction of the rectus femoris muscle, a two joint muscle that crosses both the hip and the knee joints. Its action is to flex the hip and extend the knee.[31]

With the patient prone, flex the knee fully. At this point, a tight rectus femoris will cause the patient to lift the buttocks off the table. In patients with L4 root irritation, pain will occur in the quadriceps muscle.

13. Check reflexes. In clinical neurology, the distinction is made between lesions of the upper motor neurons and those of the lower motor neurons.

Upper motor neuron lesions present the following signs and symptoms: 1. paresis (incomplete loss of muscle power) or paralysis, 2. initial loss of muscle tone followed in time by spasticity, 3. increased deep tendon reflexes and 4. positive Babinksi sign. The lower motor neuron lesions present the following signs and symptoms: 1. paralysis of muscles innervated by these axons or their fibers, 2. decreased muscle tone, or flaccidity, 3. atrophy of muscles and 4. diminished deep tendon reflexes.

Achilles reflex, or ankle jerk. In lesions of the S-1 nerve root, the ankle reflex is diminished or absent. Both sides are tested. The patient lies supine with knee on involved side flexed at 90 degrees and the ankle jerk is then tested. There is wasting of calf muscle as well.

The gluteus maximus is also innervated by S-1 root. To test this muscle the patient is asked to raise the buttocks off of the exam table five to ten times. If there is weakness of this muscle it will be seen on this test, as the buttock of the affected side is weaker and the patient will find it difficult to raise that buttock after the first few times.

Patellar tendon reflex. L4 root lesions cause weakness of the quadriceps muscle. Note the girth of this muscle 5 inches from the upper pole of the patella and compare the affected side with the unaffected side. In addition, the patella reflex on the affected side is absent or diminished compared to the unaffected side. The girth of the quadriceps muscle on the weak side is less than the unaffected side at 5 inches from the upper pole of the patella. **Babinski's** sign. Stroke the sole of the patient's foot along the lateral border using a blunt instrument. The normal reflex is plantar flexion of the toes. When the response is dorsiflexion of the great toe and ankle with abduction of the toes, the sign is positive.

This test must be performed if an upper motor neuron lesion is suspected. If the sign is positive, the patient must immediately be referred back to the physician for prompt attention. In an adult, the sign indicates compression of the cord or inter-cranial pyramidal tract disease. See Figure 32.

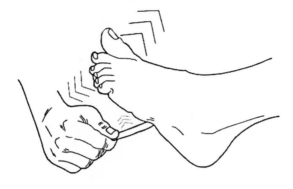

Positive Babinski's Test
Figure 32

14. **Non-organic, or functional evaluation.** When the patient's subjective complaints are not borne out by objective findings, physical therapists must be aware of other aspects of the problem. Psychological and socioeconomic factors, including litigation involving monetary gain, may be involved. Physical therapists must be aware of these aspects of the problem. A few observations can confirm the non-organic, or functional character of the case, then the patient must be referred back to the original physician with the caution that an expert mental health evaluation is needed. This senior author uses the following criteria:

   1.   Watch the way the patient moves from chair to treatment table. Grimaces and theatrical expressions are clues, but by themselves are not definitive.

   2.   This author performs another SLR test, this time with the patient in the sitting position. If the patient tolerates having the leg raised to 90 degrees without pain, when the test from the supine position did elicit pain, this is suggestive of non-organic pathology.

3. If, at the end of the SLR test, the foot is plantar-flexed rather than dorsiflexed and the patient complains of pain, he may be malingering.

Waddell describes[32] five signs which are not highly sensitive nor specific to evaluate these patients and some authors[33] proclaim that they merely identify patients with neuropathic pain. Caution is advised with these patients. Signs of functional illness do not rule out major organic pathology. Both mental and physical illness may be involved. But the patient's psychological problems and anxieties both about the back and about working must be fully explored or many back problems can become chronic despite physical treatment. For a full discussion of chronic back pain, see chapter 7.

ADDITIONAL TESTS TO CONFIRM THE DIAGNOSIS

Various diagnostic tools newly available to the physical therapist can facilitate accurate diagnoses of intervertebral disc disease and other mechanical disorders of the lumbar spine.

CT Scans can aid in diagnosing the problem during the acute stages of strain/sprain. Acute intramuscular injuries appear as areas with low electron density, an indication of inflammation.

MR Imaging. The study of tendons, ligaments, muscles and the previously invisible collagen is now possible with MR Imaging using the Magic Angle or other solid-state imaging techniques such as short-echo time.[34]

Back muscle fiber in patients with low back pain may differ from those in normal persons. The trunk muscles, due to their dual function of maintaining stability of the vertebral column and controlling intervertebral spinal motions, have a better capacity for endurance than do other muscle groups. Nicolaisen et al.[35] attribute this to the mainly Type I fibers of which they are composed. Ranging from 49-67%, Type I fibers are slow-twitch oxidative fibers characterized by slow contraction and extremely high endurance. In patients with low back pain, however, the dominant fiber is a different type, Type II, these authors postulate. Hultman et al.[36] found, by using both isometric tests and MRI, that patients with chronic low back pain had less extensor strength and endurance and lower density in their erector spinae muscles than normal subjects.

Serum creatine kinase is seen at high levels, about five times greater than normal, in patients with acute muscle injuries, according to Malone.[37] Lieber[8,39] has shown that eccentric muscle activity can cause or increase creatine kinase levels, but this may not strongly correlate with either muscle pain or the magnitude of muscle injury.

X-rays cannot be used to diagnose disc disorders or other causes of nerve irritation. They are mainly used to evaluate fractures, instability, tumors, abnormal motion and other bony details that can be clearly seen on them.

CT with myelogram has been replaced by MRI, and is used only when the patient has a Pacemaker or other metal implant. When combined with a myelogram, the CT scan provides valuable information about the nerve roots.

ELECTROMYOGRAPHY AND SURFACE ELECTRO-MYOGRAPHY (EMG & SEMG)

Both of these test the functions of the nerve roots and the way they affect muscle function. They help differentiate neuropathy from radiculopathy (nerve-root compression). By inserting needle electrodes into muscles, we can study the muscles' electrical activity at rest and on volition. Surface EMG, on the other hand, uses surface electrodes attached to the superficial muscles. EMG and SEMG are mainly used for patients with low back pain to evaluate the direct relationship between muscular pain and increased electrical signals over normal resting levels.

TESTS FOR DISC HERNIATION IN PATIENTS WITH SCIATICA

Various tests for lumbar disc herniation among patients with sciatica have estimated accuracies as follows:

Test	Sources	Sensitivity	Specificity
Ipsilateral SLR	Kosteljianitz et. Al. 1984 Hakelius et al 1972	0.80, 0.40	+ leg pain at 60°
Crossed SLR	Spangfort, 1972 Hakelius et al 1972	0.25, 0.90	+ pain on contra-lateral leg
Ankle Dorsiflex weakness	Spangfort, 1972 Hakelius et al 1972	0.35, 0.70	HNP L4-5 80%
Weak Great Toe	Hakelius et al 1972	0.50, 0.70	HNP L5-S1 60% L4-L5 30%
Reduced ankle reflex	Spangfort, 1972	0.50, 0.70	HNP L5-S1 Absent reflex = greater specificity
Sensory Loss	Kosteljianetz, 1984	0.50, 0.60	Poor predictor of HPN

Patella reflex	Aronson et al, 1963	0.50, --	HNP upper lumbar
Weak ankle plantar flexors	Hakelius et al, 1972	0.06, 0.95	
Weak quads	Hakelius et al, 1972	<0.01, 0.99	

According to Hudgins[40], preoperative physical findings are as follows for patients with proved disc displacement.

Painful crossed SLR	97%
Weakness	90%
Asymmetric reflex	90%
Sensory deficit	70%

Various computer-aided tests for herniated lumbar discs have sensitivities and specificities determined by Hudgins as follows[41]:

	Sensitivity	Specificity
Computed tomographic scan	0.92	0.88
Metrizamid myleography	0.90	0.87
Discography	0.83	0.78
Electromyography	0.92	0.38

For diagnosing low back pain, Van den Hoogen et al. provide for the following sensitivities and specificities of various tests[42]:

Test	Sensitivity	Specificity
Sciatica	0.79, 0.91	0.14
Parasthesia	0.30, 0.74	0.18, 0.58
SLR	0.88, 1.00	0.11, 0.44
SLR 30 deg	0.12, 0.27	0.94
Crossed SLR	0.23, 0.44	0.86, 0.95
Poor ankle reflex	0.31, 0.56	0.57, 0.89

Poor patellar reflex	0.04, 0.15	0.67, 0.96
Weak great toe extensor	0.30, 0.82	0.52, 0.89

Common Conditions

In 1955, Charnley[43] described the mechanisms of intervertebral disc pathology and multiple conditions, correlating pathologic/anatomic factors with clinical presentation and treatments. White and Punjabi[44] updated Charnley's work and this senior author further modified it, covering the situations most commonly seen in physical therapy practice and the relevant treatment strategies he uses with his patients. These are, as follows:

Acute Back Strain/Sprain with
Annular fiber rupture

Clinical Picture:
1. Specific Incident: A person lifts a heavy object.
2. Acute pain in low back with referred pain to buttock.
3. Muscle spasms.
4. Negative SLR.

Treatment:
1. Rest as needed.
2. Analgesics.
3. 90/90 postion, 30 minute, 2 times daily.
4. Neurostimulation (Interferential Therapy), 15 minutes to low back.
5. Back School.
6. Cold packs/Hot packs.
7. LLLT.

8. Exercises for legs – hamstrings, glutei, quadriceps, etc.

9. Isometric back exercises after 3 weeks, within pain tolerance. Home program of 90/90, and walking in pool for 10-20 minutes, followed by breathing exercises.

Postero-Lateral Annulus Disruption:

Clinical Picture:
1. Back pain
2. Hip and upper leg pain.
3. Negative SLR.
4. No muscle weakness.

Treatment:
1. Bed rest for 2 to 3 days.
2. Analgesics.
3. 90/90 position, twice daily for 30 minutes.
4. Interferential Therapy.
5. LLLT.
6. Cold or hot packs.
7. Leg and hip exercises from third day.
8. Back exercises isometric – Isotonic within pain tolerance in 3 weeks.
9. Walking in pool daily for 10-20 minutes.
10. Home program of breathing exercises and walking daily.

Bulging Disc, Sequestrated Fragment, Displaced Sequestrum Fragment:

Clinical Picture:
1. Back pain.

2. Pain on coughing and sneezing.
3. True sciatica.
4. SLR positive.

Treatment:
1. Rest as needed.
2. Pain management.
3. Cold packs, LLLT, Interferential Therapy.
4. Cortrell Back Traction.
5. Strengthening exercises to lower extremities.
6. Back stabilizing exercises after 3 weeks when pain has subsided.
7. Back School.
8. Jacobson's Relaxation exercises.
9. Breathing exercises.
10. Home program of 90/90 position twice daily for 30 minutes and walking in pool with breathing exercises.

CHAPTER 6 NOTES

1. Delitto A, Erhard RE, Bowling RW. A treatment based classification approach to low back syndrome: Identifying and staging patients for conservative treatment. *Physical Therapy.* 1995; 75: 470-485.
2. Fritz JM. Use of a classification approach to the treatment of three patients with low back syndrome. *Low Back Pain* (APTA Monograph). 1998: 84-95.
3. Spitzer WO. Scientific approach to the assessment and management of activity-related spinal disorders: a monograph for clinicians- Report of the Quebec Task Force on Spinal Disorders. *Spine.* 1987; 12: S1-S59.
4. Wemeke M. Discriminant validity and relative precision for classifying patients with nonspecific neck and back pain by anatomic pain patterns. *Spine.* 2003; 28: 161-166.
5. American Physical Therapy Association: Guide to Physical Therapist Practice. *Physical Therapy.* 1997; 77: 1163-1650.
6. International Classification of Impairments, Disabilities, and Handicaps: a manual of classification relating to the consequences of disease. Geneva, Switzerland: World Health Organization; 1990.
7. White AA, Punjabi MM. *Clinical Biomechanics of the Spine.* 2nd ed. Philadelphia: Lippincott-Raven; 1990.
8. Chamley J. Acute lumbago and sciatica. *British Medical Journal.* 1955; 1: 344.

9. Deyo RA. Lifestyle and low back pain: the influence of smoking and obesity. *Spine.* 1989; 14:501.

10. Nachemson AL. Scientific diagnosis or unproved label for back pain patients? In: Szpalski M, Gunzburg R, Pope M, eds. *Lumbar Segmental Instability.* Philadelphia: Lippincott-Raven; 1999: 297-301.

11. Macnab, lan. *Backache.* Baltimore: Williams & Wilkins; 1978: 97-98.

12. Nachemson AL. The lumbar spine: an orthopedic challenge. *Spine.* 1976; 1:59.

13. Nelson RM, Nestor DE. 'Standardized assessment of industrial low-back injuries: Development of the NIOSH low-back atlas. *Topics in Acute Care and Trauma Rehabilitation.* 1988; 2: 16-30.

14. Waddell G, Somerville D, Hendersson I, Newton M. Objective clinical evaluation of physical impairment in chronic low back pain. *Spine.* 1992; 17: 617-628.

15. Riddle DL, Rofhstein JM. Inter-tester reliability of McKenzie's classifications of the syndrome types present in patients with low back pain. *Spine.* 1992; 17: 1333-1339.

16. Riddle DL. Classification and low back pain: a review of literature and critical analysis of selected systems. *Low Back Pain: APTA Monograph.* 1998:26-55.

17. Waddell G, Somerville D, Hendersson I, Newton M. Objective clinical evaluation of physical impairment in chronic low back pain. *Spine.* 1992; 17: 617-628.

18. Deyo RA. Rational clinical examination. *Journal of the American Medical Association.* 1992; 268: 760-765.

19. Borenstein DG, Wiesel SW, Boden SD. *Law Back Pain.* 2nd ed. Philadelphia: WB Saunders; 1995:77.

20. Mayer TG, Tener AF, Kristoferson S, Mooney V. Use of noninvasive techniques for qualification of spinal range of

motion in normal subjects and chronic low back pain dysfunction patients. *Spine.* 1984; 9: 588.

21. McKenzie RA. Prophylaxis in recurrent low back pain. *New Zealand Medical Journal.* 1979; 89:22-23.

22. Fernando CK. Letter to the editor. *Physical Therapy.* 1991; 71: 2.

23. Esses SI. *Textbook of Spinal Disorders.* Philadelphia: JB Lippincott; 1995.

24. Waddell G, Somerville D, Hendersson I, Newton M. Objective clinical evaluation of physical impairment in chronic low back pain. *Spine.* 1992; 17: 617-628.

25. Moll J, Wright V. Measurement of spinal movement. In: Jayson M, ed. *Lumbar Spine and Back Pain.* Bath, UK: Pitman; 1976: 93.

26. McCombe PF, Fairbank JCT, Cockersole BC, Pynsent PB. Reproductability of physical signs in low back pain. *Spine.* 1989; 14: 908-918.

27. Macnab I. *Backache.* Baltimore: Williams & Wilkins; 1978:123.

28. Esses SI. *Textbook of Spinal Disorders.* Philadelphia: JB Lippincott; 1995.

29. Kapandji IA. *Physiology of the Joints.* Edinburgh: Churchill Livingstone; 1974; 126.

30. Fajersztajn D. m: Borenstein DG, Wiesel SW, Boden SD, eds., *Low Back Pain* Philadelphia: WB Saunders; 1995: 95.

31. Macnab I. *Backache.* Baltimore: Williams & Wilkins; 1978: 128

32. Waddell G. *The Back Pain Revolution.* Edinburgh Churchill Livingstone; 1998: 173-240.

33. Centeno JC, et al. Waddell's Sign Revisited? *Spine.* 2004; 29: 1392.

34. Bydder GM. New approaches to magnetic resonance

imaging of intervertebral discs, tendons, ligaments, and muscles. *Spine.* 2002; 27: 1264-1268.

35. Nicolaisen T, Jorgensen K. Trunk strength, back muscle endurance and low-back trouble. *Scandinavian Journal of Rehabilitative Medicine.* 1985; 17: 121-127.

36. Hultman G, Nordin M, Saraste H, et al. Body composition, endurance, strength, cross-sectional area and density of MM erector spinae in men with and without low back pain. *J Journal of Spinal Disorders.* 1993; 6: 114-123.

37. Malone TR, Duncan PW, Garrett WE. *Muscle Injury and Rehabilitation.* Vol. 3. Baltimore: Williams and Watkins; 1988: 33.

38. Lieber RL, Woodbum TM, Friden J. Muscle damage induced by eccentric contractions of 25% strain. *Journal of Applied Pl-ysiology.* 1991; 70: 2498-2507.

39. Lieber RL, Schmitz MC, Mishra DK. Contractile and cellular remodeling in rabbit skeletal muscle after cyclic eccentric contractions. *Journal of Applied Psychology.* 1994; 77: 1926-1934.

40. Hudgins RW. Predictive value of myelography in the diagnosis of ruptured lumbar discs. *Journal of Neurosurgery.* 1970; 32: 1521.

41. Hudgins RW. Computer-aided diagnosis of lumbar disc herniation. *Spine.* 1983; 8: 604-615.

42. Van den Hoogen HMM, Koes BW, Van Eijk JTM, Bouter LM. On the accuracy of history, physical examination and erythrocyte sedimentation rate in diagnosing low back pain in general practice. *Spine.* 1995; 20: 318-327.

43. Chamley J. Acute lumbago and sciatica. *British Medical Journal.* 1955; 1: 344.

44. White AA, Punjabi MM. *Clinical Biomechanics of the Spine.* 2nd ed. Philadelphia: Lippincott-Raven; 1990.

VII

CHRONIC LOW-BACK PAIN

The number of patients whose back pain becomes chronic is large. At any given time, the number of chronic sufferers is about 6% of the adult population.[1,2]

Various kinds of chronic pain exist, depending on the presenting symptoms. Many patients' problems become chronic because either they were not properly diagnosed at the outset or they received poor treatment. Consequently, they were left with unresolved difficulties such as neural and musculoskeletal dysfunction, central sensitization of their acute pain, poor education or poor self-management.[3]

Pain that is persistent and intermittent and lasts over six months is chronic, according to IASP and others. Melzack and Wall define chronic pain as pain that begins as acute but continues after the tissues involved have healed.[4]

Pain Unrelated to Objective Findings

Waddell[5] describes persistent pain that is unrelated to tissue damage as chronic. Patients become progressively less active, with resulting disability and mood changes as their apprehensions of work and somatic difficulties lead to anger, hostility, sleep

199

deprivation and the troubles that ensue. These serious psycho-social problems are beyond the scope of this book. Patients with such problems must be referred to multi-disciplinary rehabilitation centers.

Psycho-social factors include cultural and racial influences, beliefs, and attitudes toward pain and emotional and stressful responses. All of these factors affect perception of pain either positively or negatively. The presence of psychiatric problems such as depression, anxiety, and other personality disorders affect intensity of pain.

Garchel et al.[6] were able to predict, with an accuracy of 90%, which types of patients with acute back pain would become chronic patients. Their study indicated that the individuals preexisting personality, psycho-social characteristics and socioeconomic factors are the main determinants of whether acute pain becomes chronic.

Tension Myositis Syndrome (TMS)

A change in the state of the muscle due to tension that constricts circulation, depriving the muscle of blood and thereby causing spasms and nerve pain, has been described by Sarno.[7]

Sarno's[8] treatment is based on educating patients as to the nature of the disorders so that, based on their insight and understanding, they can change their behavior.

Some patients referred for physical therapy may fall into this category and should be referred for such treatment, which is beyond the scope of this book.

Undiagnosed Disc Lesions

Many chronic pain patients suffer from disc lesions that are undiagnosed, hence they are given inappropriate treatments.[9]

Internal Disc Disruption

A 1991 study showed that 40% of chronic low back pain patients had IDD.[10] And, as mentioned, about 40% of chronic low back pain originates from the intervertebral disc.[11]

IDD is a distinct clinical entity first described by Crock[12]; it differs from other painful degenerative conditions such as degenerative disc disease. Management of IDD has been through conservative care or fusion, but a new invasive procedure known as Intradiscal Electrothermal Therapy is now being used with mixed results.

Diagnosis of IDD

History includes chronic complaints of pain in the lumbar region with concomitant buttock pain, but hardly any radiculopathy. The pain usually begins with a forceful flexion motion or with a compression force acting on the lumbar spine. Flexion, rotation or side bending of the lumbar spine aggravates the pain and rest relieves it. A major trigger of this pain is sitting.

SLR test shows no radicular pain, but may show back pain. Another complaint is of localized tenderness at the lower back on palpation. Flexion of the lumbar spine to 20-30 degrees produces pain. When asked to stand up from a sitting position, these patients do so from a fully flexed position. They complain also of muscle spasms, detectable by SEMG, limited range of flexion and loss of lumbo-pelvic rhythm. Routine radiology findings are negative with no narrowing of disc space, no osteophytes or instability. Of the MRI findings, the most sensitive is the presence of a high-intensity zone (HZ), defined as an increased signal intensity, seen within the posterior annulus on T-2 weighted images. According to April and Bogduk[13], the HIZ is a clear indication of IDD. The presence of an HIZ at the posterior annulus in combination with decreased or absent T-2 signal is positive proof of IDD. Discography, with or without CT, is a very important adjunct in the diagnosis of EDD, and according to many experts is the only way to diagnose IDD.[14, 15]

Use of CT scan is helpful in diagnosing IDD and those with radial tears of the annulus. Three types of tears are seen in the annulus: 1. A concentric tear is an oval cavity due to the disruption of short transverse fibers connecting the annular lammae. 2. A transverse tear is a rupture of the Sharpey's fibers near their attachment to the ring apophysis, and 3. A radial tear is one that extends from the nucleus to the outermost layer of the annulus. Resulting pain is correlated to radial fissures on discography.

Compression injuries from axial loading due to gravity or muscle action damage the intervertebral disc. Slipping on ice, for instance, or falling on the buttocks is a gravitational injury that can damage the disc. Pulling and lifting heavy loads can injure muscles that can impact on the disc. Any compression injury beyond a certain threshold can fracture the end plate, and ultimately the end plate heals without pain. But the fracture may propagate a disruption of the internal disc, either due to an inflammatory repair process or due to an unknown autoimmune mechanism.[16]

Deterioration of the nucleus pulposus decreases its water-binding capacity and its shock absorbency. The disc thus loses height, and a condition of isolated disc resorption ensues. The deterioration of the nucleus pulposus also has deleterious affects on the annulus, as it develops radial fissures.

HISTORY OF CHRONIC LOW-BACK PAIN

Nearly 10% of patients with acute low back pain become chronic sufferers. In a 1995 study[17], nearly 40% of chronic low back pain patients were diagnosed as having IDD, and many of these patients improved with conservative care. Another study[18] indicates that nearly 40-60% of these patients improve and the rest have worsening pain and disability.

TREATMENT OF CHRONIC LOW-BACK PAIN

During the early stages, the best results are obtained with a combination of rest, modification of activity, non-steroid anti-inflammatory medication and therapeutic exercises, mainly lumbar extension exercises with stabilization exercises, and epidural steroid injections. Since the natural history of the patient is not well-known, it is best to continue the physical therapy treatment for a minimum of 4-6 months.[19]

Physical Therapy Treatments include educating the patient in how to care for the back and management to decrease pain. This clinician uses sub-thermal doses of SWD or ultrasound with cortisone, 1.5 watts per square centimeter for 7 minutes, followed by 90/90 Cortrell traction to unload the spine and aid in the healing process. Breathing exercises and Jacobson's relaxation exercises are helpful in dealing with patients' apprehensions and fears. Patients are also advised on a home program of exercise, including, if possible, walking in a pool.

In cases where conservative care fails, Intradiscal Electrothermal Therapy (IDET) or fusion is advocated, but again, the results are not usually very satisfactory.

Strengthening Exercises are often advocated for chronic low back pain.[20] Strong evidence exists that exercises and cognitive therapy are more effective than ordinary conservative care.

In 1965, while working at New York University on a Fulbright Fellowship, this senior author was the first therapist in the U.S. to advocate the use of flexion, extension and iliopsoas strengthening exercises to stabilize the lumbar spine. At that time, these concepts were not accepted. The other physiatrists at Rusk Rehabilitation Institute would not allow Fernando to treat their patients, but the mentor with whom he worked, Dr. John Sarno, believed in him and had the courage to refer patients to Fernando for therapy. These patients then became the subjects of the comparative studies that comprised Fernando's Masters' Thesis at NYU in 1969 and papers presented at two international conferences.[21, 22] Now, of course, the whole world has accepted these concepts.

Chronic low back pain patients have more atrophy of back extensor muscles and psoas muscles than do normal persons. These patients are less strong generally, according to many studies.[23, 24] The effects of an exercise program are: 1. A gain in muscle strength because of neural drive, 2. An increased density due to hypertrophy of the muscle fibers and 3. An increased cross-sectional area.

Cognitive intervention is simply counseling patients to understand that regular exercise is helpful and that ordinary activities cannot harm the disc or the back. Cognitive therapy, along with exercises, is more effective than routine care alone. This clinician not only advises patients but also shows them a film on back care and ADL and gives them a book, *Fight Back,* that covers these matters and explains exercises and the proper use of the back.

CHAPTER 7 NOTES

1. Croft PR, Papageorgiou AC, Thomas E, et al. Short term physical risk factors for new episodes of low back pain. Prospective evidence from the South Manchester Back Pain Study. *Spine.* 1999; 24: 1556-1561.

2. Croft PR, Papageorgiou AC, Ferry S, et al. Psychological distress and low back pain. Evidence from a prospective study in the general population. *Spine.* 1995; 20: 2731-2737.

3. Braggins S. *Back Care: A Clinical Approach.* Edinburgh: Churchill Livingstone; 2000.

4. Melzack R, Wall P. *The Challenge of Pain.* Harmondsworth: Penguin; 1996.

5. Waddell G, Main CJ. A new clinical model of low back pain and disability. In: Waddell G, ed., *The Back Pain Revolution.* London: Churchill Livingstone; 1998.

6. Gatchel RJ, Polatin PB, Mayor TG. The dominant role of psycho-social risk factors in the development of chronic low back pain disability. *Spine.* 1995; 20: 2703-2709.

7. Sarno J. *Mind Over Back Pain.* New York: Berkeley Books; 1986.

8. Sarno J. *Healing Back Pain.* New York: Warner Books; 1991.

9. Grubb SA, et al. The relative value of lumbar roentgenograms, metrizamide, myelography, and discography in the assessment of patients with chronic low back syndrome. *Spine.* 1983; 12: 282-283.

10. McCoy CE, Selby D, Henderson R, Handal J, Peloza J, Wolf C. Patients avoiding surgery: Pathology and one year life

status follow-up. *Spine.* 1991; 16: S198-S200.

11. Schwarzer AC, Aprill CN, Derby R, et al. The prevalence and clinical features of internal disc disruption in patients with chronic low back pain. *Spine.* 1995; 20: 907-912.

12. Crock HV. Internal disk disruption. A challenge to disc prolapse fifty years on. *Spine.* 1986; 11: 650-653.

13. Aprill C, Bogduk N. High intensity zone: A diagnostic sign of painful lumbar disc on magnetic resonance imaging. *British Journal of Radiology.* 1992; 65: 361-369.

14. Holt EP. Question of lumbar discography. *Journal of Bone Joint Surgery.* 1968; 50: 720-726.

15. Weinstein J, Claverie W, Gibson S. Pain of discography. *Spine.* 1988; 13: 1344-1348.

16. Bogduk, N, Twomey L. *Clinical Anatomy of the Lumbar Spine.* Melbourne: Churchill Livingstone; 1970.

17. Smith SE, Darden BV, Rhyne AL, Wood KE. Outcome of un-operated discogram-positive low back pain. *Spine.* 1995; 20: 1997-2001.

18. Lanes TC, Gauron EF, Spratt KF, Wernimont TJ, Found EM, Weinstein JN. Long-term follow up of patients with chronic back pain treated in multi-disciplinary rehabilitation program. *Spine.* 1995; 20: 801-806.

19. Lee C, et al. In: Fardon DF, Garfin SR, Abitol J, et al. (Eds.) *Orthopedic Knowledge Update: Spine.* American Academy of Orthopedic Surgeons; 2002; 35.

20. Van Tulder MW, Matauvaara A, Esmail R, Koes BW. Exercise therapy for low back pain: a systematic review within the framework of the Cochrane collaboration back review group. *Spine.* 2000; 25: 2784-96.

21. Fernando CK, Sarno JE. Low back pain. A new rationale and technique of treatment by therapeutic exercises. *Proceedings of the First International Assembly.* Asian Pacific League of

Physical Medicine; 1970.

22. Fernando CK. Treatment of low back pain. *Proceedings of the World Confederation for Physical Therapy: 7th International Congress;* 1974.

23. Parkkola R, et al. Magnetic resonance imaging of the discs and trunk muscles in patients with chronic low back pain and healthy control subjects. *Spine. 1993;* 18: 830-836.

24. Reid S, et al. Isokinetic trunk-strength deficits in people with and without low back pain: a comparative study with consideration of effort. *J Spinal Discord.* 1991; 4: 68-72.

VIII

PHYSICAL THERAPY TECHNIQUES

The purpose of physical therapy is threefold: 1. to reduce pain and spasms, 2. to increase strength, endurance, flexibility, and range of motion, and 3. to counsel patients on resuming their ordinary activities and preventing re-injury.

REDUCING PAIN AND SPASMS

Laser Therapy

(Light Amplification by Stimulated Emission of Radiation). Laser application for photobiostimulation in physical therapy is presently known as low-level laser therapy (LLLT). It has been used in Europe, Japan and Canada for about 20 years, yet the U.S. Food and Drug Administration has allowed LLLT in physical therapy practice only in the last few months.

This senior author uses a gallium-aluminum-arsenide (GaAlAs) semiconductor, or diode laser, for pain management. This has had excellent results. Minimizing pain and inflammation also accelerates the healing process. The unit used is an 810nm, 1W laser diode infrared probe.

The Rationale for Using Laser Therapy

The postulated physiological and therapeutic action of LLLT is as follows: Chromophores (skin pigments that are light-absorbing molecules such as melanin) absorb the photons. The LLLT thus induces a photobiomodulation effect on biological tissues, manifested as a photochemical reaction. A high dose triggers a cellular-photoinhibition response used to manage pain. A low dose triggers a cellular-photobiostimulation response that enhances tissue healing.[1] LLLT irradiation increases proliferation of satellite cells, the precursor cells in muscle regeneration.[2] And LLLT can increase collagen production in connective tissue and soft-tissue injuries by increasing the intra-and-inter-molecular hydrogen bonding in the collagen molecules, thereby improving tensile strength. This also accelerates healing.[3]

Much controversy surrounds the effects of LLLT on pain. Some studies have shown a significant change (increase/decrease) in the distal conduction latencies of the median and radial nerves after LLLT treatment.[4,5] Others, however, have shown no such effect.[6] Bashford[7] found the use of laser on low back pain to have good results, and Tarn[8] found its use on low back pain (ankylosing spondylitis) to have fair results.

Another study, by Fung et al.,[9, 10] found that using the Ga-Al-As laser significantly enhances the ultimate tensile strength, stiffness, and collagen fibril size of surgically repaired medial collateral ligaments. Studies by Weiss[11] and Bibikova[12] found that in the skeletal muscle of rats and toads, He-Ne laser irradiation of injured sites enhanced regeneration of skeletal muscle by two- and eightfold, respectively, relative to non-irradiated controls. Several studies show that low level laser therapy is effective in relieving pain from several musculoskeletal conditions including tendonitis[13], shoulder injuries[14], myofasciitis[15], fibromyalgia[16], calcaneal spur[17], carpal tunnel syndrome[18,19], osteoarthritis[20,21] and rheumatoid arthritis.[21] While studying the effects of pain, Baxter et al.[22] reported that lasers achieved the premier overall ranking for pain relief compared with the other electro-physical modalities. A rapid relief from neck pain[23] as well as back pain[24,25] has been reported by several investigators following laser application.

CRYOTHERAPY

During the acute stage, cold is more beneficial than heat according to various studies.[26,27,28] Another study, however, indicated the opposite: heat was more beneficial during the acute stage.[29] So if cold packs provide no relief for a particular patient in the acute stage, heat may be tried.

Ice packs may be applied to the affected muscle or ligament for 10 minutes every 6 hours. But cryotherapy must be discontinued if it causes neuropathic pain and aggravation of edema. If beginning cryotherapy relieves pain and causes no vascular changes, it may be continued, but not prolonged indefinitely because this could cause permanent nerve damage.

The Rationale for Using Cold Therapy is that the resulting arterial vasoconstriction minimizes bleeding, so that less fluid infiltrates the interstitial tissues. In addition, by lowering metabolism and decreasing vasoactive agents such as histamines, cold therapy reduces inflammation. Less pain and fewer muscle spasms result.

The flip side of this is that repetitive and prolonged ice application can damage myelinated sensory and motor nerves. Prolonged ice application, according to Moeller et al.,[31] can lead to hardening and solidification of the lipid-rich myelin sheath, and this can cause transient paralysis of the motor and sensory nerve fibers for as long as one year.

The authors of the Cochrane review[32] isolated three studies involving a total of 179 patients with osteoarthritis on the knee. In one of these studies, patients given ice massage were compared with a control group not receiving ice massage. The patients who received ice massage improved more than the control group in range of motion and strength.[32]

ULTRASOUND (US)

Various studies validate the use of Ultrasound (US) during the acute stage. Along with cryotherapy, US is a treatment of choice during the first 24-72 hours for all muscle strains and for ligamentous sprains Grades 1 and 2. It may also be an adjunct treatment for surgically-treated Grade 3 ligamentous sprains.

The patient must remove all clothes above the waist other than a surgical gown and lie prone with a pillow under the abdomen. This exposes the area to be treated so that US can be directly applied to the muscle or ligament, about 1-1.5W/sq cm for 7 minutes. Following the procedure, the patient is advised to rest as completely as possible to avoid aggravating the injury and to enhance the healing process.

US penetration is greatest up to 2 inches below the surface, causing significant heating.[33] In addition, there is evidence that US also has non-thermal effects resulting from vibration of the molecules, which increases membrane permeability and allows increased ionic exchange.

The Rationale for Using Ultrasound. Recent animal studies show that low intensity US accelerates the healing of spinal fusion after treatment with muscle pedicle bone grafts.[34] The healing is aided in several stages: gene expression, blood flow, tissue modeling and remodeling. These findings may be extrapolated to the repair of human muscles, tendons and ligaments.

In a recent study, 60 patients with osteoarthritis of the knees were treated either with US or with phonophoresis with ibuprofen.[35] Researchers found no difference in efficacy of the two treatments. Patients in both groups showed significant gains in pain scores and range of motion. Patients and physicians alike were satisfied with both modalities.

DEEP FRICTION

In addition to cryotherapy and US, deep friction to the affected muscle, ligament or musculotendinous junction can be helpful during the acute stage of strains and sprains, i.e. for the first seven days.

In muscle strains, deep transverse friction separates adhesions between individual muscle fibers that restrict movement, thereby mobilizing the muscle. If the patient follows up such passive mobilization by adequate active use of the muscle, a cure will be effected since the adhesions cannot then reform.[36]

In ligamentous sprains, the early application of deep friction disperses blood clots or effusions. By moving the ligament back and forth over the subjacent bone in imitation of its movement during normal use, mobility is maintained and the ligament is numbed enough to facilitate active movement later on.[37]

SUPERFICIAL HEAT

Hot packs at temperatures of 77°C (170°F) can be applied for 20 minutes at each therapy session during the later stages of strains and sprains. Benefits are due to increased blood flow and hyperemia, according to Lehman et al.[38] Superficial heating with hot packs reduces muscle spasms by decreasing gamma-efferent activity, which lowers alpha motoneuron activity.[39]

INTERFERENCE CURRENT THERAPY (ICT)

In addition to its use for pain reduction, ICT can be used for reeducating, strengthening and relaxing muscles. Electrode placement over spinal nerve roots for analgesic purposes is more effective for patients with acute than for those with chronic low back pain.[40]

Two electrical currents with different frequencies, one 4000 hertz and the other 4100 hertz, are applied to the skin through surface electrodes. This ensures that an interference pattern is established at the intersection of the two currents. As a result, the targeted tissue receives a low frequency of 100 hertz, which helps depolarize motor and sensory nerves. Thus deep stimulation of muscle and nerve is possible at lower frequencies of 1-10 hertz and this can be used for muscle reeducation, strengthening and relaxation. In addition, smooth muscles surrounding blood vessels respond well to stimulation at these lower levels, so this technique can be used to treat patients with reflex-sympathetic dystrophy (RSD). Noble et al.[41] showed that ICT produced a significant increase in blood flow to the quadriceps muscles in healthy subjects.

MANIPULATIVE THERAPIES

Any therapy not based on sound clinical judgment can do the

patient more harm than good. One has only to look at studies advocating manipulation and mobilization to see the dangers to which some therapists expose their patients. In a study by Fritz et al. advocating manipulations for patients with low back pain or numbness in the lumbar spine buttock or lower extremity, the authors admit they do not know what tissues are affected by their techniques. Despite this, they claim there are hardly any risks involved in lumbar manipulation.[42] A study[43] published by the UCLA School of Public Heath indicated that results of chiropractic care and medical care for low back pain were comparable after six months and that the possible benefits of physical therapy are small, but may be marginally more effective than medical care alone for reducing disability of some patients.

Nachemson[44] reports that inconsistent findings make it impossible to judge whether manipulation is more effective for acute low back pain than other applications such as massage, short-wave-diathermy and exercises or such drugs as analgesics or NSAIDS, but he states that manipulations should not be used in cases of patients with serious or progressive neurological problems in view of the serious, but rare neuralgic complications.

Spinal manipulation may be defined as dexterous, passive movement of a joint within or beyond its active range of motion, and may vary from the traditional, forceful thrust to oscillation and distraction.[45] The technique has been performed on patients with low back pain since ancient times and was described by Hippocrates in 400 B.C. Lately, its popularity has grown, and more physicians, physical therapists, osteopaths and chiropractors are adopting it in their practices.

It is generally known that manipulation can exacerbate low back pain and even cause injuries.[46] Despite the need for adequately controlled clinical trials to evaluate manipulation, the medical literature on the subject, until the 1970s, consisted merely of descriptions of the technique and reports of cases or uncontrolled series. In an interesting 1969 study[47], Matthews and Yates used epidurography to show that manipulation reduced the size of the small disc protrusions of two patients, an effect not previously demonstrated. But no other treatments, only control maneuvers, were employed for comparison.

In the first controlled clinical trial of rotational manipulation of the trunk, 84 British industrial workers suffering from low back pain were randomly allocated into two groups.[48] One group was given one lumbar rotational manipulation and four daily simulated diathermy (placebo) treatments. The other group was given five daily simulated treatments. Interestingly, patients in both groups, whether their pain was of recent origin or of a month's duration, reported a rapid, marked improvement immediately after the study began and continuing over a seven-day period. The manipulated patients, however, reported slightly greater pain relief in the first fifteen minutes after the first treatment.

Other investigators also have reported positive effects of manipulations, but their studies have been criticized on the grounds that they did not take into account the strong placebo effect of the "laying-on-of-hands" and did not employ appropriate controls for comparison.

In 1981, Hoehler, Tobis and Buerger[49] reported on a clinical trial comparing the results of spinal manipulations with the results of a sham treatment, a soft-tissue massage that patients could not distinguish from the manipulation technique. Of their ninety-five patients, fifty-six were given spinal manipulation as follows: The patient lay on his/her side facing the practitioner, with the lower leg extended, the upper leg flexed, the upper side of the pelvis tilted toward the practitioner and the upper side of the shoulder titled away from him. The practitioner then made a quick, brief thrust to open the joints of the lower back and stretch the muscles. The thirty-nine control patients were given only the soft-tissue massage. Subjective evaluations were confirmed by measurements of straight-leg raising to pain, straight-leg raising to pelvic rotation[50] and distance of the fingertips from the floor on maximum forward flexion.[51] But by the time the patients were discharged, all had substantially improved, and those given spinal manipulation reported no greater improvements than those given only the massage. Hoehler et al.[52] concluded that spinal manipulation gives immediate subjective relief of low back pain, but there is no evidence that it affects the long-term outcome.

In 1984, Godfrey et al.[53] published the results of a controlled clinical study of 81 patients with acute low back pain. Rotational manipulation of the trunk was compared to two other procedures, namely minimal massage and low-level electro-stimulation, which the authors considered unlikely to have any effect. All patients, those who received manipulation and those who received the control treatments, improved rapidly during the period under study. Initial and final assessments were made on scales quantifying symptoms, activities of daily life, mobility, tenderness to palpation, aggravation of pain by coughing or sneezing, limitation of motion and forward flexion. The authors found no difference between the improvement of the patients who received the manipulation and those who received the control treatments. Godfrey et al." point out the many problems involved in performing and analyzing controlled studies: recruitment of patients is slow; delays occur in diverting patients into a study group; the dearth of patients makes randomizing difficult; a large number of patients are needed to preclude Type II error, i.e. incorrectly concluding that there is no real difference between two observed groups (that the manipulation treatment has no real efficacy); manipulation may not always be the same because styles vary among practitioners; investigators must depend upon

216

patients' subjective reports of immediate effects; they must depend upon patients' cooperation in making measurements; and appropriate placebo treatments must be devised that will not bias patients' evaluations. Finally, these authors urge caution in interpreting the reports of previous investigators that manipulation helps patients with acute low back pain of recent onset.

Spinal mobilization involves low-velocity, passive movements within or at the limit of joint range. The guidelines of the United States (AHCPR) and United Kingdom support the use of spinal manipulation, at least with patients with acute low back pain. But this study, done after these guidelines were issued, came to an entirely different conclusion- "In the meantime, we conclude that the efficacy of manipulation for patients with acute low back pain has not been convincingly demonstrated with sound RCTs."[54] They also go on to say that the efficacy of manipulation has not been established for chronic conditions either.

Since this study few other studies have been documented and results have been mixed. In all these other studies the RCTs were of poor quality, with heterogeneous groups of patients.[55] The complications of spinal manipulations are not too well documented. Yet those that are documented are enough evidence not to use this modality in any practice. "Do manipulations harm the patient? The answer is yes, sometimes."[56] Nachemson[57] indicated after a thorough literature search that there is no clinically significant proof that manipulation for acute or subacute low back pain is superior to bed rest and salicytates.

After reviewing the literature, we believe it possible that patients with specific disorders may be helped by manipulation. If so, this group deserves to be precisely identified by a randomized, large-scale study of a population with a wide range of histories. We believe, further, that MRI scans should be made before and after the manipulation to verify that the procedure returned something that was out-of-place to a more normal position. MRI scans also should be made of patients receiving other treatments, placebo treatments, and no treatment, for comparison. In short, *the efficacy of manipulation should be proved before it is made a standard procedure.*

In the meantime, we must be mindful of the dangers involved in manipulative therapies and the potential harm they can do. Particularly vulnerable are patients with an acute disc, neurologic signs, spondylosis, fracture or joint instability.[58]

We must remember, too, that most patients do not need extreme and controversial measures; they will improve in time with the most conservative treatments. Some improve even with no treatment. So the careful, conscientious practitioner will continue to favor conservative treatments. These measures should be tried before any drastic procedures such as manipulation, traction, chemonucleolysis, or surgery are undertaken.

INCREASING STRENGTH, ENDURANCE, FLEXIBILITY AND RANGE OF MOTION

Exercises

Isometric and Isotonic Exercises can be started when the patient is comfortable enough, usually 2-3 days after cryotherapy, US and deep friction treatments. The patient must perform the exercises while lying down on a stable, flat surface (not a ball). Isometric exercises are given first, then isotonic.

Strength, Endurance and Flexibility Exercises

Once the patient's pain and spasms have abated, usually after 7-10 days, strength, endurance and flexibility exercises may be started.

Range of Motion Exercises

If pain and spasms are not first resolved, trying to increase range of motion is an exercise in futility. Passively stretching any structure must not be attempted. With increasing performance of isotonic strengthening exercises, the patient automatically increases range of motion. Machines to develop strength and endurance also enhance range.

The Rationale for Strengthening Exercises

A ligamentous spine isolated and fixed at its base would collapse under a force of only 4.5 lbs.[59] The fact that it usually does not collapse during normal daily activities is due to the functioning of two systems that stabilize the lumbar spine, namely the extrinsic and intrinsic stabilizers. The extrinsic stabilizers of the lumbar spine are composed of all the muscles surrounding it. The intrinsic stabilizers are the ligaments and intra-abdominal pressure. Thus the need is to strengthen the abdominal, extensor and iliopsoas muscles. Strengthening the abdominal and back extensor muscle groups not only strengthens the extrinsic stabilizers, it also increases the integrity of the intrinsic stabilizers: intra abdominal pressure opposes, and so minimizes, the forces on the lumbar spine. And by streghtening theiliopsoas, the extrinsic stabilizers are also strengthened. As a further indication that strengthening the iliopsoas is necessary, this group of muscles is seen to be weakened in patients with low back pain.[60]

The concept of strengthening the extrinsic and intrinsic stabilizers is not new. The senior author, C.K. Fernando, has successfully used the technique in his practice since 1966.

Other authorities, too, have documented the benefits of strengthening exercises. Hides et al. [61] compared two groups having a first episode of acute low back pain. One group was given medication and advice and the second group was given exercises to strengthen the transverse abdomonis muscle and the multifidus. The recurrence rate 2-3 years later was 75% for the medically managed group compared to only 35% for the group given exercises. An earlier study by Hides et al.[62] showed that even after ten weeks of treatment, the multifidus does not return to its normal size. This may contribute to the high recurrence rates after an acute episode of low back pain, as a large portion of patients may have a deficit in their lumbar stabilizing capacity despite the absence of pain, as these authors point out.

Further validation for the efficacy of exercises is the fact that they are the most commonly used treatment in clinical practice. A study by Mielenz et al.[63] indicated that 83% of patients were given exercises, 74% heat, 65% US, 50% electrical stimulations, 49% massage, 35% cold packs, 21% spinal manipulation and adjustments, 16% traction and 6% other treatments for low back pain.

Since the physical therapy exercises outlined in this book strengthen the abdominal, extensor and iliopsas muscles, they are more effective than exercises that strengthen only the abdominal muscles such as Williams' flexion exercises or those that stretch the lumbar spine such as McKenzie's extension exercises. Moreover, manipulations and mobilizations by themselves treat the joints, not the muscles and ligaments, therefore are inappropriate in the treatment of strains and sprains of the lumbar spine or any other back conditions. The exercises are given to low back patients to strengthen their muscles, thereby stabilizing the spine; any exercise that causes pain must not be used. All exercises are within the patient's pain tolerance.

There is widespread disagreement regarding various exercise systems and guidelines. Some authorities use exercises for patients with low back pain: 1. To strengthen abdominal and back muscles and increase flexibility; 2. To enhance blood flow to the muscles, joints and discs, thus minimizing injury and promoting repair; and 3. To improve the patient's mood and thereby lessen the perception of pain.[64] Nachemson believes that exercises are the most preventative intervention, even though most studies that indicate this were methodologically flawed.[65]

The latest System Review on Exercise Therapy for Low Back Pain[66] concluded that for acute low back pain, exercise was no more effective than inactive or active treatments. For chronic low back pain, exercise therapy was more effective than usual care by the general practitioner and just as effective as conventional physiotherapy.

Under these circumstances clinicians should continue the safest and best-result oriented practices unless a particular technique proves far superior to others in a specific case.

It is safest not to mobilize or manipulate the back; the rest of currently advocated treatments should be continued until we can be certain what the best treatments are.

Traction/Distraction

Traction is a drawing, or pulling force, as along the long axis of a structure. Distraction is a drawing apart. Pelvic traction and lumbar traction have been used to treat patients with low back pain since ancient times, even before Hippocrates.

Many therapists and physicians have employed many traction and distraction techniques to spaces between the discs, to decompress the discs and increase the inferior-superior dimensions of the intervertebral foramina. This allows more space for the spinal nerve roots, arteries and veins. In other words, it decompresses the structures that are compressed.[67] In addition, traction improves the blood supply to soft tissues in the posterior part of the spine as well as the vertebral end plates, thereby increasing the blood supply to the disc, which helps in the diffusion of oxygen and nutrients in to the disc.

The Cortrell distraction system involves suspending the patient over a stool with knees and hips bent at 90 degrees. A rope attached to a belt around the patient's pelvis is draped over the top of a triangular frame. The therapist or patient can pull on the rope to lift the patient up by the pelvis off the stool. This technique can be used in the hospital, outpatient department or at the patient's home. It is simple and inexpensive compared to similar pieces of equipment such as the VAX-D system or the distraction reduction stabilization (DRS) system. See Figures 33 and 34.

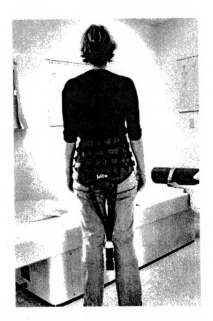

Patient with harness with VAX-D Unit in background.

222

Figure 33

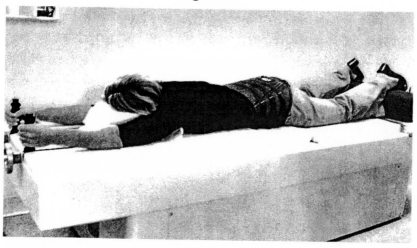

Patient in Traction in a VAX-D Unit

Figure 34

The Rationale for Traction/Distraction

We hypothesize that with use of Cortrell distraction techniques, the intradiscal pressure is reduced to negative level. This also enhances diffusion of oxygen and nutrients into the disc, promoting aerobic metabolism, which fosters biophysical functions and cellular repair activity.[68, 69] Using a VAX-D table, intradiscal pressures can be lowered to -150 to -160 mm of Hg. This is the only traction/distraction device of which this can truly be said. We believe the Cortrell system does this for the simple reason that during distraction, the paraspinal muscles are completely relaxed as our SEMG studies show. It has also been shown that lower intradiscal pressure may reduce bulging of nuclear material.

According to Cotrel,[70] the originator of this system, it provides relief to 97% of acute and 94% of chronic low-back patients. The senior author, having used this system for nearly twenty years, agrees with this assessment. Patients with lumbar

223

pain syndromes experience not only symptomatic improvement, but also improvement in magnetic resonance imaging (MRI) findings compared to pre-treatment. MRI clearly shows disc herniation reduced, disc-height increased and re-hydration of the disc after sessions of treatment within a seven week period. See Figures 35, 36, 37, 38, 39, 40, 41, 42 and 43.

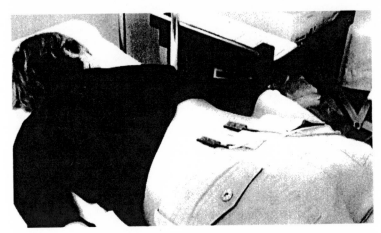

Patient in prone position with surface EMG electrodes on low back.

Figure 35

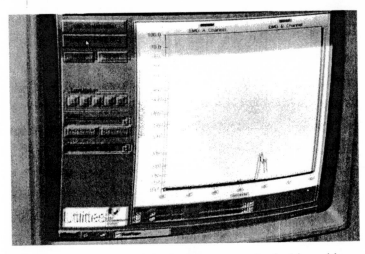

Monitor showing no activity in extensor muscles in this position.

Figure 36

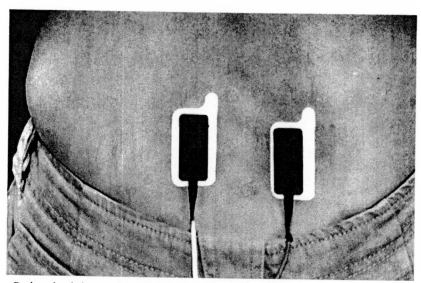

Patient in sitting position with surface EMG electrodes on extensor muscles.

Figure 37

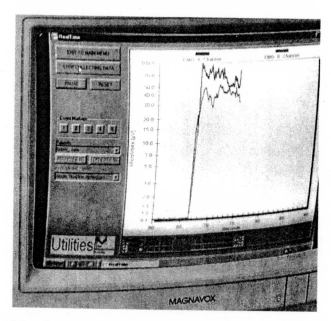

EMG activity of extensor muscles of patient in sitting position appears on monitor.

Figure 38

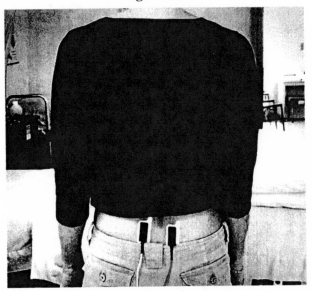

Surface EMG electrodes applied to low back of patient in standing position.

Figure 39

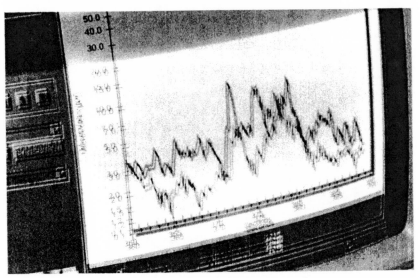

EMG activity seen in both channels.

Figure 40

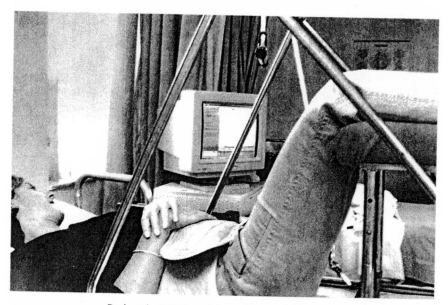

Patient in 90/90 position with no traction.

Figure 41

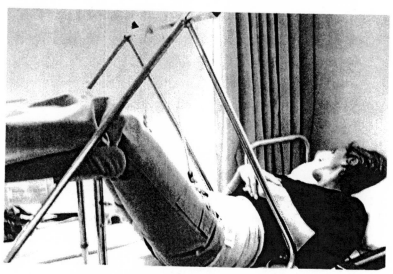

Patient in 90/90 position with Cotrell Traction.

Figure 42

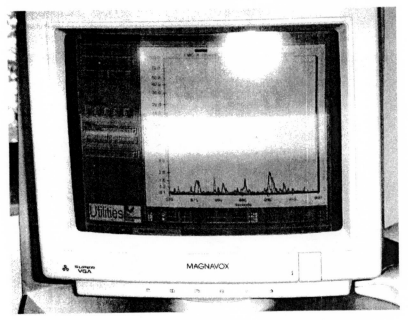

This position yields no EMG activity on monitor.

Figure 43

COUNSELING PATIENTS ON RESUMING NORMAL DAILY ACTIVITIES

Overcoming Anxieties

Most patients can be helped to confront and overcome anxieties, and this author has adopted the following strategies for the purpose in his clinical practice: For the past 25 years, a Back School film had been shown to all patients and each is given a book that details the same points. Patients are also counseled that their problem, whether a sprain, strain, or disc herniation, will resolve and the healing process is explained. They are given a home program of exercises, such as walking inside or outside a pool, breathing, and others. Chronic patients are taught Jacobson's relaxation exercises[71]. All of these measures help the

228

patient cope with their fears and continue with the rehabilitation process.

There are no safe and effective shortcuts or substitutes for the process of arriving at a diagnosis. An unscientific new therapy advocated by George et al.[72], called fear-avoidance therapy, is based on false premises. Treatment decisions are made based on only two or three symptoms with no diagnostic tests or confirming clinical imaging and radiological testing. The authors apparently generalize information gleaned from studies of chronic low back pain by Vlaeyen JW, et al.[73], and incorrectly apply this to patients with acute back pain. George's study is severely flawed in another respect as well: One group of patients, a "Standard Care" group, was given a pamphlet emphasizing anatomy and pathology. Another group, a "Fear-Avoidance" group, was given a pamphlet emphasizing the view of back pain as common, not a serious disease, and de-emphasizing anatomic findings. But both of these different aspects of back pain are valid, and for the past 35 years patients in this author's practice have been made aware of both, with good results.

Correct Use of the Back

In order to competently and effectively advise a patient, the therapist must carefully analyze the cause and mechanism of the injury. The ergonomics of the daily work environment and the patient's manner of performing accustomed routines must be investigated so that any needed corrections or modifications can be advised.

For athletes, their training and exercise programs must be evaluated and any necessary changes advised in their practices and techniques.

A Regular Exercise Program

A regular exercise program consisting of daily repetitions of the exercises described herein will continue to strengthen the muscles that support and maintain the back and to stretch and relax the ligaments around the joints of the back, making them more limber and flexible. Since a large portion of patients, despite the absence of pain after treatment, remain deficient in their lumbar stabilizing capacity, and since this factor certainly contributes to the high rate of recurrence of low back pain, it is very important that they continue with the exercise program.[74]

Motivation

Patients' motivation to practice the correct use of the back at work and at home and to continue the daily exercise program, unfortunately, may languish or disappear once an episode of low back pain has resolved. The therapist must emphasize the high rate of recurrence and the need to make a habit of correct use of the back and encourage all patients to perform the daily exercises to maintain a healthy back. If this counseling is neglected, patients are likely to re-injure themselves, entailing more severe consequences.

CHAPTER 8 NOTES

1. Reynesdal AK, Bjomland T, Barkvoll P, Haanaes,HR. The effect of soft laser application on post operative pain and swelling: a double blind cross-over study. *Intern J of Oral and Max Surgery.* 1993; 22: 242-245.

2. Shefer G, et al. Low Energy laser irradiation promotes the survival and cell cycle entry of skeletal muscle satellite cells. *Journal of Cell Science.* 2002; 115:1461-1469.

3. Enwemeka CS and Reddy GK. The biological effects of laser therapy and other modalities on connective tissue repair processes. *The Journal of Laser Therapy.* Vol. 12. World Association of Laser Therapy. 2000.

4. Basford JR, Hallman HO, Matsumoto JY, Moyer SK, Buss JM, Baxter GD. Effects of 830nm continuous laser diode irradiation on median nerve function in normal subjects. *Laser Surgery Medicine.* 1993; 13: 597-604.

5. Lowe AS, Baster GD, Walsh DM, Alien JM. The effect of low-intensity laser (830nm) irradiation upon skin temperature and antidromic conduction latencies in the human median nerve. Relevance of radiant exposures. *Lasers Surgery Medicine.* 1994; 14: 40-46.

6. Greathouse DG, Currier DP, Gilmore RL. Effects of Clinical Infrared laser on-superficial radial nerve conduction. *Physical Therapy.* 1985; 65: 1184-1187.

7. Basford JR, Sheffield CJ, Harmsen WS. Laser Therapy: A

randomized controlled trial of the effects of low intensity Nd/Yag laser irradiation on musculo-skeletal back pain. *Archive of Physical Medicine Rehabilitation.* 1999; 80: 647-652.

8. Tam G. Low-power laser therapy and analgesic action. *Journal of Clinical Laser Medical Surgery.* 1999; 17: 29-33.

9. Fung DT, Ng GY, Leung MC, et al. Therapeutic low-energy laser improves the mechanical strength of repairing medial collateral ligament. *Lasers Surg Med.* 2002; 31: 91-96.

10. Fung DT, Ng GY, Leung MC, et al. Effects of a therapeutic laser on the ultra-structural morphology of repairing medial collateral ligament in a rat model. *Lasers Surg Med.* 2003; 32:286-293.

11. Weiss N, Oron U. Enhancement of muscle regeneration in the rat gastrocnemius muscle by low-energy laser irradiation. *AnatEmbryol.* 1992; 186: 497-503.

12. Bibikova A, Oron U. Promotion of muscle regeneration in the toad gastrocnemius muscle by low-energy laser irradiation. *AnatRec.* 1993; 235: 374-380.

13. England S, Farrell AJ, Coppock JS, et al. Low power laser therapy of shoulder tendonitis. *Scandinavian Journal of Rheumatology.* 1989; 18: 427-431.

14. Calderhead G, Ohshiro T, Itoh E, et al. The Nd-YAG and Ga-Al-As lasers; a comparative analysis in pain therapy. *Laser Accupuncture.* 1982; 21: 1-4.

15. Ceccherelli F, Altafini L, Lo Castro G, et al. Diode laser in cervical myofascial pain: a double-blind study versus placebo. *Clinical Journal of Pain.* 1989; 5: 301-304.

16. Gur A, Karakoc M, Nas K, et al. Effects of low power laser and low dose amitriptyline therapy on clinical symptoms and quality of life in fibromyalgia: a single-blind, placebo-controlled trial. *Rheumatology International.* 2002; 22: 188-193.

17. McKibbin LS, Downie R. A statistical study on the use of the infrared 904-nm low energy laser on calcaneal spurs. *Journal of Clinical Laser Medical Surgery.* 1991; 9: 71-77.

18. Padua I, Padua R, Moretti C, et al. Clinical outcome and neurophysiological results of low power laser irradiation in carpal tunnel syndrome. *Laser Medicine Science.* 1999; 14: 196-202.

19. Weintraub *MI.* Noninvasive laser neurolysis in carpal tunnel syndrome. *Muscle Nerve.* 1997; 20: 1029-1031.

20. Ozdemir F, Birtane M, Kokino S. The clinical efficacy of low-power laser therapy on pain and function in cervical osteoarthritis. *Clinical Rheumatology.* 2001; 20:181-184.

21. Brosseau L, Welch V, Wells G, et al. Low lever laser therapy for osteoarthritis and rheumatoid arthritis: a metaanalysis. *Journal of Rheumatology.* 2000; 27: 1961-1969.

22. Baxter GD, Bell AJ, Alien JM, et al. Low lever laser therapy: Current clinical practice in Northern Ireland. *Physiotherapy.* 1991; 77: 171-178.

23. Airaksinen 0, Airaksinen K, Rantanen P. Effects ofHe-Ne laser irradiation on the trigger points of patients with chronic tension in the neck. *Scandinavian Journal of Applied Electrotherapy.* 1989; 4: 63-65.

24. Gur A, Karakoc M, Cevik R, et al. Efficacy of low power laser therapy and exercise on pain and functions in chronic low back pain. *Lasers SurgMed.* 2003; 32: 233-238.

25. Basford JR, Sheffield CG, Harmsen WS. Laser therapy: a randomized, controlled trial of the effects of low-intensity Nd:YAG laser irradiation on musculoskeletal back pain. *Archive of Physical Medicine Rehabilitation.* 1999; 80: 647-652.

26. Landen BR. Heat or cold for the relief of low back pain? *Physical TJierap)'.* 1967; 47:1126.

27. Hayden CA. Cryokinetics in an early treatment program. *Journal of the American Physical Therapy Association.* 1964; 44: 990.

28. Grant AE. Massage with ice (cryokinetics) in the treatment of painful conditions of the musculoskeletal system. *Arch Phys Med Rehabil.* 1964; 45:233.

29. Landen BR. Heat or cold for the relief of low back pain? *Physical Therapy.* 1967; 47:1126.

30. Hooshang H, Halshmi M, Phillips EM. Cryotherapy can cause permanent nerve damage: a case report. *American Journal of Pain Management.* 2004; 14: 63-70.

31. Moeller JL, Monroe J, McKeag DB. Cryotherapy -induced common peroneal nerve palsy. *din JSports Med.* 1997; 7: 212-216.

32. Brosseau L, Yonge KA, Robinson V, Marchand S, Judd M, Wells G, Tugwell P. Thermotherapy for treatment of osteoarthritis. *Cochrane Database SystRev.* 2003; 4:CD004522.

33. Draper DO, Castel JC, Castel D. Rate of temperature increase in human muscle during 1 MHz and 3 MHz continuous UltraSound. *Journal of Orthopedic Sport Physical Therapy.* 1995; 22:142-150.

34. Aynaci O, Onder C, et al. The effect of ultrasound on the healing of muscle-pediculated bone graft in spinal fusion. *Spine.* 2002; 27: 1531-1535.

35. Kozanoglu E, Basaran S, Guzel R, Guler-Uysal F. Short term efficacy of ibuprofen phonophoresis Versus continuous ultrasound therapy in knee osteoarthritis. *Swiss Med Wkly.* 2003; 133:333-338.

36. CyriaxJ. *Textbook of Orthopedic Medicine.* 10th ed. London: Bailliere Tindall; 1980: 13.

37. Cyriax J. *Textbook of Orthopedic Medicine.* 10th ed. London: Bailliere Tindall; 1980 : 14.

38. Therapuetic Heat. In: Lehmann JF, ed. *Therapeutic Heat and Cold.* 4th ed. Baltimore: Williams & Watkins- 1990.

39. Physiological responses to heat and cold. In: Licht S, ed. *Therapeutic Heat and Cold.* 2nd ed. Baltimore: Waveriy Press; 1965.

40. Hurley DA, Minder PM, et al. Interferential therapy electrode placement technique in acute low back pain: a preliminary investigation. *Arch Phys Med Rehabil.* 2001; 82: 485-493.

41. Noble JG, Henderson G, et al. The effect of interferential therapy upon cutaneous blood flow in humans. *Clin Phsyiol.* 2000; 20: 2-7.

42. Fritz JM, Erhard RE, Hagen BF. Segmental Instability of the Lumbar Spine. *Physical Therapy.* 1998; 78: 889-896.

43. Hurwitz EL. A randomized trial of medical care with and without physical therapy. *Spine.* 2002; 27: 2193-2204.

44. Nachemson AL. A critical look at the treatment for low back pain: The research status of spinal manipulative therapy. DHEW Publication. 1975; No (NIH) 76-998: 21B.

45. Koes BW, Assendelft WJ, van der Heijden GJ, Bouter LM. Spinal manipulation for low back pain. An updated systematic review of randomized clinical trials. *Spine.* 1996; 21: 2860-2871.

46. Sims-Williams HJMIV, Young SMS, Baddeley H, Collins E. Controlled trail of mobilization and manipulation for patients with low back pain in general practice. *British Medical Journal.* 1978: 1338-1340.

47. Mathews JA, Yates DAH. Reduction lumbar disc prolapse by manipulation. *British Medical Journal.* 1969; 179: 696-697.

48. Glover JR, Morris JG, Khosia T. Back pain: A randomized clinical trial of rotational manipulation of the trunk. *British Journal of Industrial Medicine.* 1974; 31: 39-64.

49. Hoehler FK, Tobis JS, Buerger AA. Spinal manipulation for low back pain. *Journal of the American Medical Association.* 1981; 245: 1835-1838.

50. Fisk JW. The passive hamstring stretch test: Clinical evaluation. *New Zealand Medical Journal.* 1979; 89: 209-211.

51. Doran DML, Newell DJ. Manipulation in the treatment of low back pain: A multi-center study. *British Medical Journal.* 1975; 2: 161-164.

52. Hoehler FK, Tobis JS, Buerger AA. Spinal manipulation for low back pain. *Journal of the American Medical Association.* 1981; 245: 1835-1838,

53. Godfrey CM, Morgan PP, Schatzker J. A randomized trial of manipulation for low back pain in a medical setting. *Spine.* 1984; 9: 301-304.

54. Koes BW, Assendelft WJ, van der Heijden GJ, Bouter LM. Spinal manipulation for low back pain. An updated systematic review of randomized clinical trials. *Spine.* 1996; 21:2860-2871.

55. Shekelle PG, Adams AH, Chassin MR, Hurwitz EL, Park RE, Phillips RB, et al. The appropriate use of spinal manipulation for back pain: indications and ratings by a multi-disciplinary expert panel. Santa Monica, CA; 1991

56. White AA, Punjabi MM. *Clinical Biomechanics of the Spine.* 2nd ed. Philadelphia: Lippincott-Raven; 1990: 441.

57. Nachemson AL. A critical look at the treatment for low back pain: The research status of spinal manipulative therapy. DHEW Publication. 1975; No (NIH) 76-998: 21B.

58. Paris SV. Spinal manipulative therapy. *Clinical Orthopaedics and Related Research.* 1983; 179:55-61.

59. Morris JM. Role of the trunk in the stability of the spine. *Journal of Bone and Joint Surgery.* 1961; 43A: No. 3.

60. Fernando CK: Treatment of low back pain: Review of recent research findings with rationale and technique of treatment. *Proceedings of the World Confederation for Physical Therapy, 7th International Conference.* 1974.

61. Hides J, et al. Long term effects of specific stabilizing exercises for first-episode low back pain. *Spine.* 2001; 26: E243-E248.

62. Hides J, et al. Multifidus muscle recovery is not automatic after resolution of acute, first-episode low back pain. *Spine.* 1996; 21: 2763-2769.

63. Mielenz TJ, Carey TS, Dyrek DA, et al. Physical therapy utilization by patients with acute low back pain. *Phys Ther.* 1997; 77: 1040-1051.

64. Nachemson A. *Neck and Back Pain.* Philadelphia: Lippincott; 2000: 140.

65. Nachemson A.. *Neck andBack Pain.* Philadelphia: Lippincott; 2000; 145.

66. Van Tulder MW, Malmivaara A, Esmail R, Koes BW. Exercise therapy for non-specific low back pain. *Spine.* 2000; 25: 2784-2796.

67. Colachis SC, Strohm BR. Effects of intermittent traction on separation of lumbar vertebrae. *Arch Phys MedRehabil.* 1969; 50: 251-258.

68. Anderson, G-, Schultz, A, Nachemson, A-Intervertebral Disc Pressure During Traction. *Scand. Journal of Rehabilitation Medicine.* 1968; 9: 88-91.

69. Mathews JA. Dynamic discography: a study of lumbar traction. *Ann Phys Med.* 1968; 9: 275-279.

70. Cortrell 1981

71. Jacobson E. *Progressive Relaxation.* Chicago: University of Chicago Press; 1938.

72. George SZ, Fritz JM, Bialosky JE, Donald DA. The effect of

a fear avoidance-based physical therapy intervention for patients with acute low back pain: Results of a randomized clinical trial. *Spine.* 2003; 28: 2551-2560.

73. Vlaeyen JW. Fear of movement/re-injury in chronic low back pain and its relation to behavioral performance. *Pain.* 1995; 62: 363-372.

74. Hides J, et al. Long term effects of specific stabilizing exercises for first-episode low back pain. *Spine.* 2001; 26: E243-E248.

IX

A PLEA FOR PROGRESS

The most important challenges now facing those of us who study low back pain are:

1. To establish the most reliable and efficient clinical techniques for diagnosis and treatment as the standard for the profession. This will assuage the anxieties of patients and doctors alike.

2. To increase understanding of episodic, non-specific backache.

3. To postulate a better theory explaining such episodes in order to replace the present, competing theories, which breed rival and conflicting treatments, frustrate patients and damage clinicians' credibility.[1]

DEFINITIVE DIAGNOSES USING STANDARD TERMINOLOGY

To achieve these aims, first of all, all professional personnel involved in the treatment must use the same standard medical terminology. We must use the same vocabulary, speak the same language, if we are to effectively communicate with each other.

At the present time, the majority of centers caring for back patients use one label, namely LBP, for all patients with low back pain, and treat them all the same way. This oversimplification may well be a major factor in the recent explosion of back surgeries in the U.S. Because there are many different kinds of back problems, there is no one-size-fits-all therapy. This must become well understood.

Diagnoses of all back problems must be standardized using the age-old accepted methods of allopathic medicine, beginning with a history and a clinical examination followed by any appropriate tests, such as laboratory and radiological tests (X-ray, MRI, CT Scan, EMG and Spinex), to clarify or confirm the clinical diagnosis.

In addition, all personnel, whether physicians or physical therapists, must use anatomical terms as defined by the *Nomina Anatomica,* physiological terms accepted by the relevant scientific group and the diagnostic system according to the ICD. Only if all professions involved in the treatment process use the same scientific and medical definitions of terms can we understand each other and communicate effectively. Standardization of diagnostic techniques and the language used to describe back problems will go a long way toward facilitating the entire treatment process and improving the final outcome for the patient.

METHODOLOGY FOR RESEARCH STUDIES

If research studies are to be meaningful, here, too, the subjects must be given an accurate diagnosis using standard terminology instead of being classified along with other back patients as though they all had the same disease. All research into low back pain will be dramatically enhanced when the patients are accurately classified as having sprain, strain, spondylosis, disc herniation, spinal stenosis, spondylolisthesis, etc. At the present time, however, nearly all published non-surgical intervention studies of low back pain have included all categories of back pain in one group and so have reached erroneous conclusions. Some Scandinavian experiments, if performed on patients in the U.S., would be cause for malpractice suits.

Various authors present physical therapy studies as if they are scientific when they are not randomized, controlled or double-blinded. As a case in point, the study by Deyo et al.[2] set out to study acupuncture-like effects of TENS (transcutaneous stimulation), yet used frequencies in the 20-30 hertz range! Other technical flaws were the diversity of the patient population and problematic randomization. Traction studies also contain similar methodological errors including a too small subject population so that the conclusion, that traction is ineffective, cannot be supported. The most that can be said is that we do not yet know the answer. Our retrospective study remains unpublished.

SUMMARY

The system of allopathic medicine relies on tests, both specific and sensitive, to arrive at a diagnosis based on pathology. Many physicians and therapists advocate this time-tested system based on pathoanatomic, neurophysiologic, bio-chemical factors and psychosomatic factors, along with the rational use of diagnostic studies where needed to confirm the clinical diagnosis. The disease is then treated with physical therapy based on sound diagnosis and with methods proved reliable in clinical practice or research. We cannot emphasize strongly enough the fact that the most common reason for surgery is the poor quality and failure of conservative care.[3]

CHAPTER 9 NOTES

1. Deyo RA. Low back pain - a primary care challenge. *Spine* 1996;21:2826-2832.

2. Deyo RA, et al. A controlled trial of transcutaneous stimulation (TENS) and exercises for chronic low back pain. *New England Journal of Medicine.* 22: 1627-1634.

3. Marquardt C A, et al. Clinical Presentation and Diagnostic Subsets. Cole H, ed., *Low Back Pain Handbook:* A Guide for the Practicing Clinician. Second Edition. 2003; Hanley and Belfus, Inc: 95-115

APPENDIX A

EXERCISES FOR LOW BACK PAIN

FOREST HILLS INSTITUTE

FOR BACK PAIN

EXERCISES FOR LOW BACK PAIN

GENERAL INSTRUCTIONS

All exercises done:
1. On bed with board, or on floor
2. Within limits of pain
3. Three times a day, each exercise performed 3 times, progressing up to 10 times.

Always allow adequate time for exercise program. *Never rush.* Keep breathing.

Starting position – Supine Lying
1.
   a. Raise head to look at toes
   b. dorsiflex
   c. press knees to bed

Hold for count of three and relax slowly

2.

a. Arch back, only shoulders and buttocks to rest on bed. Hold for count of three and relax slowly.

b. Press your lower back down into the floor by tightening your buttocks and abdominal muscles. This is a *pelvic tilt*.

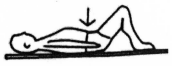

Starting position – Prone lying

3. Raise head, hold for count of three and lower slowly and relax.

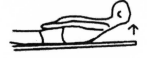

4. Raise legs alternately, first right then left with knees extended. Hold for a count of three, then lower slowly and relax.

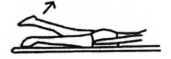

5. Clasp hands behind back, raise head and shoulders together. Hold for count of three, then lower slowly and relax.

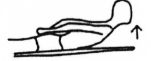

Starting position – Prone Lying

6. Hips flexed at 45°, feet held on bed by therapist or under heavy furniture. With your hands stretched towards knees, curl trunk about mid range, hold for count of three, then lower slowly and relax.

246

Starting position – Prone lying

7. With your hands by your side, raise head and shoulders together, hold for a count of three, then lower slowly and relax.

8. With your hands behind your neck, raise your head and shoulders together. Hold for a count of three, then lower your body slowly and relax.

9. With your hands extended sideways, raise your head and shoulders together. Hold for a count of three, then lower slowly and relax.

10. With your hands above your head, elbows close to your ears, raise your head and shoulders together. Hold for a count of three, then lower slowly and relax.

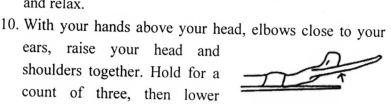

11. Pinch buttocks, then raise both legs together with knees extended. Hold for a count of three, then lower slowly and relax.

12. Combine 10 and 11. With your hands above your head and elbows close to your ears, raise your head and shoulders together. Pinch your buttocks, raise both legs together with knees extended hold combined position for a count of three, then lower slowly and relax.

Supine Lying

This exercise is to be done *only* in the clinic *with* the therapist.

13. Patient flexes hip and knee while the therapist resists movement at the knee throughout the range. At full hip flexion, the patient attempts to hold position while the therapist pulls toward extension.

APPENDIX B

MECHANICAL LOW BACK PAIN

	Muscle Strain	Herniated Nucleus Pulposus	Osteoarthritis	Spinal stenosis	Spondylolisthesis
Age (years)	20-40	30-50	>50	>60	20
Pain pattern location	Back (unilateral)	Back (unilateral)	Back (unilateral)	Leg (bilateral)	Back
Onset	Acute	Acute (prior episodes)	Insidious	Insidious	Insidious
Standing	←	→	←	←	←
Sitting	→	←	→	→	→
Bending	←	←	→	→	←
Straight leg	—	+	—	+ (stress)	—
Plain x-ray	—	—	+	+	+

INDEX

A

Achilles reflex, 106, 186

acute low back pain, 90, 105, 153, 154, 203, 214, 216, 217, 220, 221, 235, 237, 238

ADL, 21, 204

Agency for Health Care Policy and Research, ii, 2, 4, 105, 153, 217

allopathic, 7, 161, 163, 240, 241

American Physical Therapy Association, 7, 162, 195, 196, 234

annular ruptures, 17

annulus fibrosus, 17, 18, 25, 26, 76, 136

anterior longitudinal ligament, 43, 45, 65

anterior shear force, 34

anterior translation, 58, 64, 70

aortic aneurism, 2

articular processes, 15, 16, 21, 54, 55, 61, 67, 69

avascular, 17, 138

axial compression, 63, 66, 67

axial distraction, 63

axial rotation, 34, 55, 63, 66, 69, 70, 77, 100

B

back pain, i, ii, iv, 1, 2, 4, 5, 6, 7, 8, 9, 10, 11, 30, 31, 50, 52, 63, 65, 67, 68, 70, 81, 83, 85, 88, 89, 95, 97, 98, 101, 103, 106, 109, 117, 118, 119, 124, 126, 127, 130, 156, 157, 162, 164, 165, 166, 182, 188, 190, 195, 196, 199, 201, 206, 210, 229, 232, 233, 236, 243

bulging disc, 57, 94

burst fracture, 71

C

chemical radiculitis, 19

chondrocytes, 17

chronic low back pain, 2, 4, 30, 50, 189, 196, 197, 201, 203, 204, 205, 206, 207, 213, 221, 229, 233, 238, 243

clinical evaluation, iii, 7, 79, 95, 153, 161, 168, 170, 196, 197

coactivate, 31

coactivation, 47

co-activation, 27

co-contraction, 135

D

E

F

M

N

O

P